· Manual of ·
PEDIATRIC PHYSICAL
DIAGNOSIS

■

· Manual of ·

PEDIATRIC PHYSICAL

DIAGNOSIS

Lewis A. Barness, MD

Visiting Professor
Department of Pediatrics
University of Wisconsin
Madison, Wisconsin

Sixth Edition
with 57 illustrations

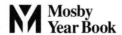
Mosby
Year Book

St. Louis Baltimore Boston Chicago London Philadelphia Sydney Toronto

Mosby
Year Book
Dedicated to Publishing Excellence

EDITOR: Stephanie Manning

EDITORIAL ASSISTANT: Colleen Boyd

PROJECT MANAGER: Carol Sullivan Wiseman

PRODUCTION EDITOR: Linda McKinley

BOOK DESIGN: Julie Taugner

COVER PHOTOGRAPH: Trustees of the British Museum, London, England

Sixth edition

Mosby–Year Book, Inc.
11830 Westline Industrial Drive,
St. Louis, MO 63146

Library of Congress Cataloging in Publication Data

Barness, Lewis A.
    Manual of pediatric physical diagnosis / Lewis A. Barness.—6th ed.
        p.   cm.
    Includes index.
    ISBN 0-8151-0494-4
    1. Children—Medical examinations.   2. Children—Diseases-
-Diagnosis.   3. Physical diagnosis.   I. Title.
    [DNLM: 1. Diagnosis—in infancy & childhood.   WS 141 B261m]
RJ50.B3   1991
618.92′00754—dc20
DNLM/DLC   91-15458
for Library of Congress   CIP

CL/MV   9   8   7   6   5   4   3   2   1

TO MY FIRST PEDIATRICIANS,
my mother and father,
AND TO
Elaine

FOREWORD

I T HAD A carnival atmosphere about it. Imagine! Medical Grand Rounds as a kind of side show! If I hadn't been there and seen it myself . . . well, let me tell you about it.

Dawkins had found a medical student, a sort of freak idiot savant, so to speak, and he was bent on displaying this boy's talents to the medical center at large. The university was rife with rumor. The boy could read minds; he was clairvoyant, psychic, and more. Dawkins had reportedly given private demonstrations of the boy's powers, thereby adding to the gossip.

The great amphitheater was packed to the plumbing fixtures—full professors down in front, students high in the rear, and all gradation of academic achievement between, layered in eight or so Dantean ledges (or circles, depending on your point of view). One could spy secretaries and laboratory technicians meekly tiptoeing in from the rear exits to stand shyly, arms folded, in the shadows. The audience hushed as Dawkins took the podium.

"Ladies and gentlemen, colleagues . . . and students, I am thrilled to present to you . . ." (Dawkins was indeed quite puffed up about this—he had always wanted to discover something).

". . . Mr Larry Tripe. Larry is a fourth-year student and, as you may have heard," Dawkins chuckled an aside, "has some special gifts to show us."

A shy young man in wrinkled white pants and a tunic entered from the left, obviously intimidated by the fanfare. He smiled self-consciously and gave a brief nod to the audience. From the opposite side of the stage Dawkins led a middle-aged man who wore pajamas, a bathrobe, and slippers. He sat the man down in the only chair on stage.

"Now Tripe . . . er, Larry," Dawkins said, eyes to the audience, "you have ten minutes. And, ladies and gentlemen, I assure you, Larry

From Lacombe MA: A piece of my mind: the cabalist, JAMA 259:3045, 1988.

has had no prior knowledge of our patient, Mr Sampson, or of his data-base."

Tripe approached the patient, shook his hand, and at the same time felt the man's radial pulse with the fingers of his left hand. He knelt on one knee before Sampson and studied the man's hands—his palms, his nails, the texture of his skin. Next he palpated the patient's neck, tilting the man's head to one side, and taking some time in doing so. The audience shifted restlessly. Tripe's face allowed a brief smile. He put an ear before the man's nostrils and seemed to listen carefully, then smiled again. He stood up, glanced self-consciously at the audience, and fumbled in his tunic's pocket, withdrawing—yes—it was indeed a stethoscope. Murmurs raced up and down the rows of the amphitheater.

Tripe gently parted the man's robe and pajama top and listened to his chest quite intently. I noticed that he had kept his fingers on the man's carotid. Tripe straightened and nodded to Dawkins, coiling the stethoscope into his pocket again. Seven minutes had elapsed.

"What you have witnessed, ladies and gentlemen, is a brief example of physical diagnosis," said Dawkins. "Well, Larry, what have you to tell us?"

"This patient has . . . well, it seems to me . . . I can hear . . . he has aortic regurgitation, sir."

Dawkins flashed the patient's catheterization data on the screen. The audience buzzed in amazement. From the front row, Professor Edgerly silenced the snickering from the students in back with an icy stare. He then turned back to Tripe and asked pointedly, "How did you arrive at your conclusion, young man?"

"Well, sir," said Tripe, "he has Corrigan's and Quincke's pulses—they're easy enough to find—and I could hear Bozzolo's sign—so I just *knew* I'd hear an aortic regurgitant murmur with my . . . with this . . . stethoscope."

Edgerly asked, "Where did you learn about these pulses and signs . . . and where did you get the stethoscope?"

"From books, sir," said Tripe. "They aren't on the computer disks. I found some old books on physical diagnosis." (Tripe had avoided, I noted, answering the second part of Edgerly's question.)

"Why in God's name," roared Edgerly, "in this age of CT scanners and magnetic resonance imaging, have you wasted your time with learning physical diagnosis?"

"It's fun, sir," replied Tripe, "and, sir, it's cheaper?"

Edgerly stood up and glared at the boy. "One requires testing to comprise a database, to diagnose, to determine course and prognosis.

This is all very amusing, but trivial . . . passé. The penultimate diagnostic tool is the test."

"Excuse me, sir," said Tripe, pressing his luck, "but I've read of another tool, sir."

"What's that?" snapped Edgerly.

"It's called taking a history, sir."

PREFACE TO THE
SIXTH EDITION

STUDENTS AND PRACTITIONERS have asked for a new edition to include more physical signs in adolescents and in those with possible child abuse. Some of these are included, but more particularly, a new edition provides an opportunity to include signs that have been observed by those who have used earlier editions.

It is distressing to note that pediatric and perhaps adult physical diagnosis is receiving less emphasis and is practiced less than previously—a downgrading caused by the development of very excellent imaging devices and sophisticated laboratory tests. This phenomenon, I think, is an error that will be compounded in the near future.

For centuries, doctors recognized the effectiveness of "laying on of the hands." When the stethoscope was invented in the nineteenth century the doctor was removed from directly touching the patient when examining the heart, lungs, and abdomen. As this phenomenon has increased, doctors may soon not confront the patient—only the computer. The distant doctor-patient relationship can only deteriorate further as the curative ability of the personal laying on of the hands disappears.

Mapping of the genome is on the horizon. Physicians will be expected to become conversant not only with diagnosis but also with prognoses and inheritability. The determination of any one person's genetic composition will be not only unbelievably costly but extremely time consuming. To most expeditiously and economically provide necessary information, physicians will be impugned to determine not only the body system but also the operative category of disease so that the proper costly confirmatory test can then be properly applied. Denigrating diagnostic physical examination skills at this time is also disheartening because of possible effects on younger physicians. They are the teachers of tomorrow, and if they do not practice now, they will be unable to teach later.

While anyone can learn later, effort expended now will improve care now.

Again, as with previous editions, I owe much to criticism of many. My wife, Enid, provided enthusiasm and support and the view of physical diagnosis through the eyes of an expert pediatric pathologist. Dr. John Bohn, a former resident, and Dr. John Silverio, a colleague, gave many helpful suggestions. My grandchildren Eliot, Alexandra, and Heather provided new challenges in diagnosis. And my consultant, Beverly Middleton, provided patience.

In spite of world turmoil, a better world can only be accomplished through our children. Anything to improve their care helps them and us.

Lewis A. Barness, MD

PREFACE TO THE
FIRST EDITION

THIS MANUAL ORIGINATED several years ago as a series of mimeographed notes to second-year medical students at the University of Pennsylvania Medical School. Each year, the notes on pediatric physical examination expanded as no suitable text for the course was found.

Three years ago Dean John McK. Mitchell and Dr. Paul György suggested that this material be gathered together in book form. The material has been further expanded for this purpose.

Physical examination is a discipline learned by observing and practicing; my teachers have supplied the opportunity for these observations. Especially among these are included Dr. Paul György, who taught me many tricks and fine points of examination of children; Drs. Charles Janeway and Sydney Gellis, who taught me the approach to the pediatric patient; Dr. Bronson Crothers, who taught an inimitable approach to the pediatric patient with neurologic disorders; seven classes of medical students, who gave free and sometimes pointed criticisms; and the many instructors in pediatric physical diagnosis at the University of Pennsylvania and Philadelphia General Hospital, who gave inestimable aid.

The preparation of the final manuscript would have been impossible without the aid of Drs. Joseph Stokes, Fred Harvie, David Cornfeld, Donald Cornely, and David Baker, who have generously given of their time and knowledge in correcting the manual. Sections of this manual have been improved with the aid of Dr. Richard Ellis, the Eye; Dr. Philip Marden, Ear, Nose, and Throat; Dr. Joseph Atkins, the Larynx; Dr. Robert Kaye, the Chest; Dr. Sydney Friedman, the Heart; Dr. C. Everett Koop, the Abdomen; Dr. Thomas Gucker, Orthopedics; Dr. Charles Kennedy, the Neurologic Examination; and Dr. Albert Kligman, the Skin. Miss L. Plunkett has been most cooperative in preparing many stencils and mimeographs of this material and its modifications for use by the students, and Mrs. J. White and Miss Lisa Weiss have completed the final typing.

To all these, and to many others whose particular aid cannot at this time be associated with a particular name, I wish to express my sincere thanks. And finally, I should like to thank my wife and daughter for their patience during the many revisions of this manual.

Lewis A. Barness, MD

CONTENTS

INTRODUCTION

A COMPLETE PHYSICAL EXAMINATION in a child emphasizes many characteristics that differ from those in adults. It is important to recognize these differences and also the many variations among normal children.

This is a manual of the special methods used in pediatric physical diagnosis. It is assumed that the person using it has the basic knowledge of physical examination of adults, for which many textbooks have been written. Therefore no extensive details are listed of the definition of a sign or of methods of eliciting a sign unless special methods are used in children. While the material in this manual includes only the actual physical examination, one must remember that diagnoses cannot be made by physical examination alone. Before beginning the examination, it is important that a careful and detailed history be taken of the patient and family and that this be made part of the patient's record. As the art of careful observation is learned, diagnosis by physical examination becomes easier. In the younger child from whom no history can be directly obtained, or in the child whose parents lack the ability of accurate observation, this is indeed necessary.

Examples of disease states will be given throughout the manual. At no time are these states to be considered the complete differential diagnosis of the sign given. The examples are given only to present a better understanding of the sign under discussion. The beginner may use this manual to learn to elicit a particular sign; the disease states indicated will later have meaning.

If further examples of a sign are desired, standard references are suggested. The references used freely in the development of this manual include the easily available standard pediatric texts.

There is no "routine" physical examination of a child. Each examination is individualized. Not only are there many physical differences that an examiner accustomed to adults might consider abnormal in a child, but also the variations among a group of children make the examiner more alert to the broad spectrum included in the term "normal." The physician adept at physical diagnosis in children is one who is aware of these variants.

Most of the observed variations can best be explained by the difference in growth rates of the organ systems as they occur from infancy to maturity. For example, the lymphoid tissue is relatively well developed in infancy, becomes maximally developed during childhood, and regresses to small adult proportions at puberty. The nervous system, on the other hand, is largely developed at birth and reaches almost complete adult size by the age of 5 years. The genital system, however, is infantile until puberty. These and other variations will be noted throughout the discussion of the physical examination.

A question frequently asked by the mother is, "Is my child normal?" One is rarely able at a single observation of that child to tell whether or not the child is entirely normal, though one may frequently be able to tell that the child is abnormal. Normality in pediatrics, as in statistics, is often confused with the average, and statisticians conclude that there is considerable variation from the average in any normal static population. Normality in children includes the many differences around the average of the age of the child being studied, with adequate consideration of the child's background and environment. Determining normality in an ever-changing individual is even more difficult. In conducting a physical examination, one looks for normal, variations from normal, and abnormal states. The general mental and physical state, congenital and acquired anomalies, and pathologic or disease states are determined.

The record of a complete physical examination in children has special importance not found in that of adults. This record of examination represents a report of one specific time in a childs' life when that child is continually and rapidly changing. Therefore it will be used as a basis for determining whether or not that child is growing and developing normally, according to a group of standards that are learned from books, mothers and patients. More important than a single observation of the child is the use made of this record in following the *rate* of change of the child at each subsequent examination. The rate of growth, rate of development, and indeed rate of progression of difficulties or anomalies far surpass for evaluation purposes the single examination. The single examination is valuable, of course, not only for determining acute illnesses, but also for determining for the physician, the parent, and the child the gross evaluation of the potentialities and liabilities of the child. Thus even small and apparently insignificant variants should be noted for each child so that their importance may be adequately assessed in later examination.

For example, if it is known that a particular child with nausea and vomiting was adequately examined 2 weeks before the illness and that the liver was not palpable at the time but is now palpable 2 cm below the right costal margin, attention would be directed to the liver as a possible cause of the illness. In contrast, if it were known that 2 weeks before the acute illness the child's liver was palpable, less attention would be paid to the now palpable liver. This type of notation is especially important for so-called innocent murmurs of childhood, which are notorious for their frequent change, the significance of which may take many months and many examinations to determine.

The physical examination in a child should also be a record that can be easily interpreted by other physicians. In appendix A, therefore, a form is included for recording a physical examination. Though the method of recording the physical examination is in a logical order, the examination itself is not necessarily performed in this order.

1

APPROACH TO THE PATIENT

ALL DOCTORS HAVE series of tricks of examination that they have developed with experience. With older children, cooperation may be improved by flattery of their clothes, conversations on their level, and discussions of mutual interests. For preschool children, you may reassure and distract patients with interesting objects. Frequently, a 2- to 4-year-old child will remain quiet and apparently interested if you start a pointless story, particularly about imaginary animals, and ask the child equally pointless questions about these animals. For infants, you must sometimes resort to physical measures such as sugar-feeding to keep them quiet. Even a 2-year-old child may respond to flattery, and although bribery of any kind is normally deplorable, a judiciously offered lollipop may create an everlasting attachment between patient and physician.

Usually, the examination is performed while the parent is present. If the child is frightened or clings to the parent, sending the parent out of the room usually serves only to frighten the child more. Failure of a 4-year-old or older child to cooperate reasonably well is evidence of something abnormal in your approach or in the child's past experience or personality. On rare occasions, you may ask the parent to leave the room, but this should be done before the examination begins or preferably before you enter the room for the examination. Ask adolescents if they desire a parent to be present. If not, a chaperone of the opposite sex of the physician should attend. Before beginning the examination, you should always wash your hands with warm water. This serves to cleanse and warm the hands so that the patient will not be uncomfortable. The parents also become aware of the consideration of the doctor and appreciate routine hand washing. If the mother stands at the examining table, she should be at the child's feet. You should organize your approach so that a part is examined only once.

In general, begin the physical examination using no instruments and gradually introduce the various necessary examining equipment. You can frequently make a tentative diagnosis by observing the child while in the mother's arms or while walking or standing in the room. This diagnosis can be confirmed following the thorough examination. Usually, patients are examined in a crib or on a table. The examining table or bed should be large enough so that children will have no fear of falling and high enough so that you can examine them in comfort.

Physical examinations are performed on children by taking full advantage of opportunities as they present themselves. Physicians concerned with the physical and mental habits of children realize that they must use all their wiles to establish rapport. The order of an adequate examination, therefore, is more or less determined by the child rather than the physician.

The examination is usually performed with patients in the position most suitable to them. Infants, severely ill children, or children who understand well may be conveniently examined largely in the supine position. However, a 6-month-old child may have just learned to sit up and may be anxious to demonstrate this ability. Therefore do the examination chiefly with the patient in the sitting position. Similarly, some children may prefer being examined while standing or in unusual positions, and these preferences should be respected if they will not interfere with a complete examination. It is especially important that children with respiratory distress be examined in the position of most comfort that provides the best airway, usually in a sitting or sometimes in a prone position.

An obstreperous or frightened patient, however, may reject all attempts at examination. Frequently, even this kind of patient can be examined completely while being held in the mothers' arms. This is especially the position of preference for many 1- to 3-year-old children. Other children may have the ears or mouth examined while being held by the mother (Figure 1-1). If the patient clings to the mother, the back and extremities may be examined in this position and the remainder of the examination can be done later with the patient supine. Examining the abdomen of a child in the mother's lap is usually unsatisfactory. If the mother is helping to restrain the patient, she should be told to hold the patient's hands rather than arms. If she holds the arms, the patient's hands are free to interfere with you.

Restraining the patient to examine such parts as the ears or mouth may occasionally be necessary. Place the infant's arms under the back so that the infant's weight rests on the palms. You or the mother can restrain the infant's head, and the examination can proceed.

Figure 1-1
The child is restrained in the mother's arms and the ears are examined.
(From Whaley LF and Wong DL: Nursing care of infants and children,
St Louis, 1987, The CV Mosby Co.)

Aware that the sight of many instruments may frighten the child,
most pediatricians start the physical examination with observation of the
hands and feet and then chest or abdomen. They then auscultate, percuss,
and palpate these areas and follow with the remainder of the examination.
The genitalia, femoral areas, and anus can be examined next in boys and
younger girls, but these areas are examined last in older girls. Next, it is
usually convenient to examine the head, eyes, face, and neck and then the
ears, nose, and throat. In the older girl the labia and introitus are then
examined. Blood pressure, measurements, and testing of mass reflexes
conclude the examination in the younger child. In the older child, blood
pressure and other measurements are determined first, and the examination may proceed from the head downward systematically as in the adult.
While performing the examination, it often helps if you allow the patient
to play with the instruments you are going to use or have just finished
using. When cooperation is desired for the difficult procedures, *tell* patients firmly what they are to do rather than *ask* them to do something.

Before anything frightening or painful is contemplated, tell patients
what is to be done and what is expected of them. Reserve procedures
such as examination of the head (where the instruments are stuck into the

ears and mouth) and the rectum for the end of the examination. Rectal examination is done whenever the patient has any symptom referable to the gastrointestinal tract. If children are old enough to understand, tell them that these procedures are "uncomfortable but not painful."

Any discomfort caused a patient should be for as short a time as possible. If you feel that at any time in the examination you must hurt the patient, do not tell the patient otherwise during the visit. If the child is acutely ill or hyperirritable, take little time for the amenities and proceed rapidly with the examination.

Occasionally, especially in the acutely ill patient, you may have suspicions regarding a particular diagnosis and may wish to confirm or eliminate this diagnosis before proceeding with the examination. For example, if meningitis is suspected in an infant, you may palpate the fontanel first, or if acute abdomen or congenital heart disease is suspected, you may examine the abdomen or heart first. Caution in following such a procedure is necessary. Too frequently, a relatively unimportant secondary diagnosis may be found, and you may forget to complete the examination that would reveal the primary diagnosis.

Caution must also be observed in following this procedure in children with obvious skin blemishes or other gross deformities or in those with suspected psychiatric difficulties or mental deficiency. In these children, examining first those areas in which difficulty is *not* expected avoids drawing the attention of the child or parent to the obvious difficulty.

Ordinarily, the complete physical examination should take the experienced physician no longer than 5 to 10 minutes to perform. Speed is necessary to avoid exhausting the patient. At each visit, regardless of the chief complaint or reason for the visit, a complete systematic examination should be performed and any abnormalities recorded. Few doctors miss diagnoses because of ignorance; errors are caused by careless omission of simple procedures.

During each examination the child should be completely undressed so that the entire body may be examined. If the room is cool or if the patient is modest or frightened, first one group of clothes may be removed and replaced and then another. The degree of modesty varies greatly among children, and modesty should be respected in a child regardless of age.

Above all, successful doctors caring for children must obtain genuine pleasure from examining and dealing with them. They should be friendly and unharried and must proceed with the examination with interest, patience, dexterity, and confidence. Children respond well to physicians who demonstrate confidence, and parents are more likely to accept diagnoses and treatment from physicians who are thorough.

2

MEASUREMENTS

T HE USUAL MEASUREMENTS taken at a physical examination include temperature, pulse rate, respiratory rate, height, weight, and blood pressure. For the child under 2 years of age, circumference of head, chest, and abdomen are also needed. These measurements are ordinarily taken at the end of the examination but are recorded first. Other measurements, such as chest and pelvic width, crown-rump distance, and sitting and standing height, are ordinarily not determined in the physical examination unless appropriate.

TEMPERATURE

The temperature is best taken either immediately before starting the physical examination or after it is over. Temperatures are probably of more value to parents than to physicians. If a patient is ill, one degree more or less of fever does not mean one degree more or less of disease. However, parents like to know how many degrees of fever their children have, and they are reassured if the temperature is normal.

Obtain a satisfactory routine temperature in a child under 6 years of age by placing the thermometer in the axilla or groin, putting the arm or the leg along the patient's body, and holding the arm or leg against the thermometer for 3 minutes. In general, axillary or groin temperatures are about 2 degrees lower than rectal temperatures and 1 degree lower than oral temperatures.

If a rectal temperature is desired, grease the thermometer well and insert it past the mercury bulb. Place the infant face down across the mother's lap with the legs dangling along the mother's leg. The mother holds the buttocks firmly with one hand and the arm of that hand lies firmly across the infant's back. The thermometer is inserted about 2 cm and held. The thermometer should be held by the parent or you as long as it is in place. Do not attempt to take the rectal temperature in children with rectal diseases or vulvovaginitis, and note that rectal temperatures are more frequently elevated than oral temperatures following exercise. Never take rectal temperatures with the child lying in a supine position because the thermometer will be inserted at the wrong angle, increasing the chances of breaking the thermometer or perforating the rectum.

Do not take oral temperatures until children understand what is expected of them, which usually occurs after 6 years of age. The newer electronic thermometers are rapid and accurate and can be used in any orifice regardless of the child's age.

Newborns may have an axillary temperature of 33° to 36° C. Only after 1 week is the temperature stabilized at 36° C axillary.

Fever is a manifestation of increased metabolism and may be caused by varied disorders. A body temperature of 40° to 40.5° C in a child corresponds roughly in significance to a temperature of 38.5° to 39° C in an adult. Children may have elevated temperatures normally after eating or vigorous playing, in the afternoon, or with excitement. Children up to 6 or even 8 years of age frequently get temperature elevations to 40° C with minor or major bacterial, viral, and protozoan infections; dehydration; and heat stroke. Upper respiratory infections or kidney infections in the infant or sinusitis, otitis, or prodromal stages of the infectious diseases in the older child are particular infections that may be difficult to determine on examination but frequently cause fever.

Fever may also be noted in children with brain injury, particularly cerebral hemorrhage or brain tumor, in those with maldevelopment of the brain, and in those who are unable to sweat because of poisoning (especially atropine) or ectodermal dysplasia. Transfusion reactions, intravascular hemolysis or inflammation, and sickle cell crisis may be accompanied by fever. Large daily temperature variations are sometimes noted with septicemia, liver or kidney disease, tumors, rheumatoid arthritis, Hodgkin's disease, and leukemia. Persistent low-grade temperature elevations to 39° C are seen often with rheumatic fever and other collagen-vascular disorders but may also be found in other conditions.

Temperature elevations over 40° C axillary, especially if the rate of elevation is rapid, are sometimes accompanied by seizures in young children with no other evidence of convulsive disorders. An elevation of this degree in a child who looks well, is playing, and has no obvious disease may indicate the presence of roseola infantum.

Hypothermia is usually due to chilling but is also seen in shock states. Especially in infants, however, you may frequently note a normal or low body temperature despite overwhelming infections.

PULSE

Obtain pulse rate in young infants by either palpation or auscultation over the heart and in older children by palpation at the wrist. The significance of the pulse rate, rhythm, and quality is discussed with the examination of the heart.

RESPIRATORY RATE

Obtain respiratory rate by watching, palpating, or auscultating the chest. In young children, accurate respiratory rates are obtained only during sleep. The significance of the respiratory rate is discussed with the examination of the lungs. Children with a rapid respiratory rate usually have respiratory distress or severe infection, and children with a slow respiratory rate usually are free from respiratory difficulty.

HEIGHT

Height or length of the child, together with weight, not only is a good measure of the overall growth of the child but also provides a record of the rate of growth for easy comparison with children of similar stature and age as recorded in standard charts. One prime characteristic that distinguishes a child from an adult is measurable growth, and if you note failure of growth, suspect some difficulty in the development of the child (see Appendix C).

Measure the infant supine. Hold the zero end of the tape at the infant's heel and read at the head to the nearest centimeter. Measure the older child who can stand on the scale. At this time, recording the approximate height of parents and grandparents is also valuable.

If broad allowances are made for normal variations and the child still appears abnormal in height, consider the variations in time of growth. Some children grow rapidly at one age and more slowly at another, and these growth spurts may not correspond to the average. If growth still appears abnormal, you should seek other explanations.

The most common cause of unusual growth seems to be genetic influence. Though height is not strictly inherited, tall parents tend to have taller children than short parents.

Abnormal *shortness* as determined by charts with standard deviations may be caused by any chronic disease affecting absorption or utilization of nutrients, including malnutrition, psychic disturbances (particularly deprivation), food allergy, food fads, kidney disease, heart disease, liver disease, pancreatic fibrosis, and other types of gastrointestinal disorders or anomalies. Children with mental deficiency, any hemolytic anemia, rickets, or juvenile diabetes may also be short. You may note dwarfing in children with disorders of the pituitary, thyroid, parathyroid, adrenal, or sex glands. Dwarfism may also be due to the chondrodystrophies or other diseases involving the spine, or no cause may be found.

Compare *sitting height* with total height in children suspected of being dwarfs. Sitting height is most easily determined by sitting the child on a hard surface with the back against the wall and measuring from the top of the head to the surface. Normally, sitting height accounts for approximately 70% of total height at birth and decreases to about 60% at 2 years of age and about 52% at 10 years. If the sitting height is greater than half the standing height, the patient has infantile stature; if the sitting height is approximately half the standing height, the patient has adult type stature.

The early attainment of adult body proportions occurs in children with sexual precocity and in dwarfs with Morquio's disease, mucopolysaccharidosis, or progeria. Persistently infantile stature or the late development of adult body proportions is seen in children with delayed adolescence, hypothyroidism, and some chondrodystrophies. Small children with normal body proportions for chronological age may have genetically small stature, pituitary or primordial dwarfism, or gonadal dysgenesis. Children with sexual precocity may have shortened lower extremities when they are fully mature.

Abnormally *large growth* is rare and usually follows overfeeding or overeating, perhaps of psychologic origin. It is also seen in children with mental deficiency. True gigantism caused by excess growth hormone from an overactive pituitary is very rare. Exceptional height is found in children with Marfan's or Klinefelter's syndrome, homocystinuria, and congenital contractural arachnodactyly. Measure arm span in children with unusual growth patterns by stretching their arms parallel to floor and holding the tape measure from fingertip to fingertip (Table 2-1). The span is more than 2 cm over height in children with Marfan's syndrome,

TABLE 2-1
Normal arm span minus height (cm)

Age	Girls	Boys
Birth	−2.5	−2.5
10 years	−1	0
12 years	0	+2
15 years	+1.2	+4.3

homocystinuria, and congenital contractural arachnodactyly, and the span is more than 2 cm less than height in children with bone or cartilage disorders or hypothyroidism.

WEIGHT

A child should be weighed routinely once a month for the first 6 months of life, once every 3 months for the next 6 months, twice a year for the next 3 years, and yearly thereafter. If you can not weigh a child because the child is holding the scale, say, "Hold your pants." The same considerations of growth and development applied to height also apply to weight except that because weight is a more accurate and easily obtainable measurement than height, it may indicate abnormality more quickly than height. The weight of the child should be compared with standard height-weight charts, and due allowances should be made for normal variations. Again, a single measurement tells little compared to the information obtained from serial measurements that tell whether the patient is gaining normally, too much, or too little.

Acute *weight loss* indicates acute illness, dehydration, or malnutrition, and chronic weight loss suggests chronic disease states. These include improper food or feeding; diarrhea; cystic fibrosis or other gastrointestinal disturbances, emotional difficulties; respiratory difficulty during feeding; mental deficiency; and renal, cardiac, or connective tissue diseases.

Rapid *weight gain* may indicate overhydration or edema but usually indicates overfeeding or overeating. A general overweight state (true obesity) is usually due to overfeeding or overeating with a generally discernible psychologic background but may be due to decreased activity, mental deficiency, or intracranial disorders. Rarely, endocrine disorders such as hyperadrenalism and hypothyroidism may be associated with obesity. In contrast to the obesity of overeating, these disorders are associated with retardation of linear growth.

HEAD AND CHEST CIRCUMFERENCES

In infants under 2 years of age, determine the head and chest circumferences immediately after measuring length. These measurements are ordinarily not obtained in children over 2 years of age. Measure the head at its greatest circumference and the chest at the nipple line. Both measurements are needed for comparison.

At birth the average head circumference is 34 to 37 cm and the chest is about 2 cm less. The head is usually about the circumference of the chest until the child is approximately 2 years old. After this age the chest continues to grow rapidly, while the head circumference increases only slightly. The significance of head and chest measurements is discussed in Chapter 4.

Body asymmetry may be noted. It is usually idiopathic but may be due to hemihypertrophy related to Wilms' tumor or other malignancies. In addition to these conditions, hemihypertrophy may result from vascular anomalies with increased perfusion and increased growth of the limb. Body asymmetry may also be due to hemiatrophy and associated with cerebral cortical injuries.

BLOOD PRESSURE

Blood pressure determinations in children are frequently overlooked. Forgetfulness or lack of proper equipment is the usual reason given for not obtaining a determination that may lead to the proper diagnosis.

Measure blood pressure either before the examination of the head or after the examination is complete and the child is dressing. The child should be relaxed and not crying. Compare the cuff to a balloon before applying it and allow the child to pump the cuff before it is wrapped. After wrapping the cuff snugly, the manometer is placed so that you and the child can see the "silver streak" of the mercury or the "clock" of the spring manometer. Place the bell stethoscope over the brachial artery.

The proper cuff size is no less than one-half and no more than two-thirds the length of the upper arm. Similar relative sizes are used for the thigh if leg pressures are taken. A larger cuff is difficult to apply and may give readings that are too low. A smaller cuff gives readings that are too high. The rubber bag inside the cuff must be long enough to encircle the arm completely. For the very obese, apply the cuff to the forearm and auscultate at the wrist.

Inflate the cuff higher than the expected systolic pressure and slowly deflate it. The wall of the collapsed vessel suddenly distends, producing the first Korotkoff sound—the systolic pressure. Further lowering is followed by a swishing sound, then a muffling—the fourth Korotkoff sound. Sound disappears at the fifth Korotkoff sound. Record systolic and diastolic pressures at the appearance and disappearance of Korotkoff's sounds, recognizing that fifth phase recordings tend to underestimate diastolic pressure. Determining fourth phase—muffling of the heart sounds—is less consistent. Take blood pressure annually beginning when the child is about 3 years of age.

If you cannot hear the Korotkoff sounds, you can make a rough estimate by applying the cuff in the usual manner, slowly deflating, and palpating the radial, popliteal, or dorsalis pedis arteries. The first pulsation felt is about 10 mm below the true systolic pressure. If these arteries cannot be felt, the hand, wrist, and forearm (or toes, ankle, and leg) can be elevated and tightly wrapped to exclude blood up to the point where the cuff is applied. Then inflate the cuff to a level above the suspected blood pressure. Remove the wrappings. Slowly reduce the pressure in the cuff; the first flushing noted in the hand or foot is close to the systolic pressure. Alternatively, after the cuff is applied, the Doppler effect can be used by a ray of ultrasonic energy beamed from a transducer to a blood vessel. The receptor can use earphones or an electronic recorder.

If you fail in the first attempt at obtaining the blood pressure, remove the cuff before attempting again, since even a deflated cuff may hurt or frighten the child. If you obtain an elevated blood pressure, repeat the measurement and measure the pressure in the other three extremities. In any patient suspected of having heart disease, measure the blood pressure in the four extremities.

Blood pressure at birth is about 60 to 90 mm systolic and 20 to 60 mm diastolic. Both pressures usually rise 2 to 3 mm per year of age; adult levels are reached near or shortly after puberty (Figure 2-1). Crying or apprehension may double these levels. Pulse pressure is normally 20 to 50 mm throughout childhood. Systolic pressure in the arms may equal that in the legs in children up to about 1 year of age. Thereafter the pressure in the legs should be about 10 to 30 mm higher than that in the arms. The diastolic pressure should be almost equal in the arms and legs. If it is not, the cuff size is proper for the arms but too small for the legs. Very large differences in arm and leg systolic pressures (Hill's sign) suggest aortic insufficiency.

Elevated blood pressure values (both systolic and diastolic) may be noted, especially in children with any renal disease including pyelonephritis, acute or chronic glomerulonephritis, renal artery stenosis, the nephrotic syndrome, neuroblastoma, familial dysautonomia, renal tumors, and, rarely, renal calculi. Elevated blood pressures may also be found in children with increased intracranial pressure, Cushing's disease, pheochromocytoma, neurofibromatosis, hyperthyroidism or hypothyroidism, neuroblastoma, vitamin A or D poisoning, or connective tissue diseases. Elevated blood pressure may also be found in children with bulbar poliomyelitis, usually during the acute phase of the disease. The mechanism is unknown but may be due to the loss of a depressor reflex. Spinal cord lesions also may cause hypertension. An elevated blood pressure is usually found in one or both upper extremities of children with coarctation of the aorta or thoracic aortitis.

Unequal blood pressures in the arms occur in children with the scalenus-anticus syndrome with cervical rib or with a coarctation of the aorta

Figure 2-1

Age-specific percentiles of BP measurements in **A,** Girls: birth to 12 months of age; Korotkoff phase IV (K4) used for diastolic BP. **B,** Girls: 1 to 13 years of age; K4 used for diastolic BP. (*Courtesy American Academy of Pediatrics.*)

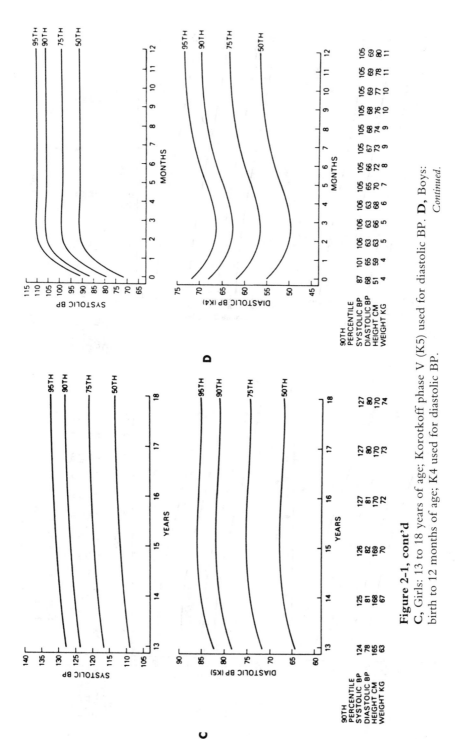

Figure 2-1, cont'd
C, Girls: 13 to 18 years of age; Korotkoff phase V (K5) used for diastolic BP. D, Boys: birth to 12 months of age; K4 used for diastolic BP.

Continued.

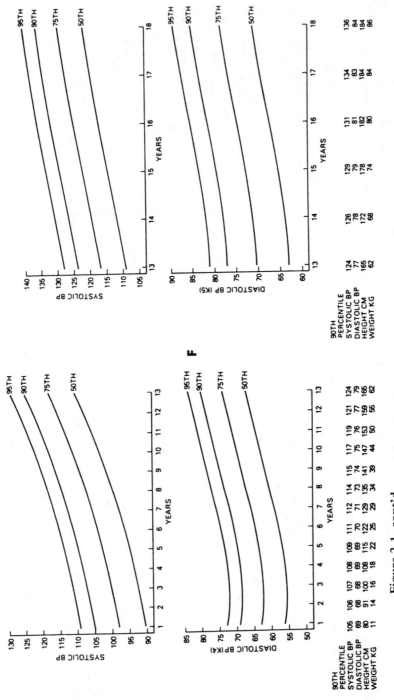

Figure 2-1, cont'd

E, Boys: 1 to 13 years of age; K4 used for diastolic BP. F, Boys: 13 to 18 years of age; K5 used for diastolic BP.

proximal to the left subclavian artery. Some children with patent ductus arteriosus have unequal arm blood pressures.

Variable systolic pressures are *pulsus paradoxus*. Inflate and lower the pressure cuff several times. Irregular or fading beats occur with inspiration. The difference between the first faint sounds and repetitive crisp regular beats (the normal systolic difference with inspiration) is about 10 mm (see Chapter 5).

Elevated systolic pressure alone or with a broadening of the pulse pressure is noted after exercise or excitement or in febrile states. It is usually seen with a lowered diastolic pressure in children with patent ductus arteriosus, arteriovenous fistula, or aortic regurgitation.

Normal or elevated diastolic pressure with a low systolic pressure, and therefore a *narrow pulse pressure,* is noted in children with aortic or

TABLE 2-2

Approximate limits for mid-upper arm
circumference and triceps skinfold

Age	Mid-upper arm circumference 3d to 5th percentile* (cm)	Triceps skinfold 90th to 97th percentile† (mm)	
		Boys	Girls
Newborn	9	10	10
3 mo	10	11	11
6 mo	11.5	12	12
9 mo	12	13	13
12 mo	13	14	14
2 yr	13	13	13
3 yr	13	13	13
4 yr	13.5	13	13
5 yr	13.5	13	13
6 yr	14	12	15
7 yr	14	13	16
8 yr	14.5	14	17
9 yr	15	14	18
10 yr	16	16	20
11 yr	16.5	17	21
12–16 yr	17–20	18–20	22–25

Modified from Zerfas AJ and Neumann CG: Office assessment of nutritional status,
Pediatr Clin North Am 24:253, 1977.
*Under this value suggests undernutrition.
†Over this value suggests obesity.

subaortic stenosis or with hypothyroidism. A widened or elevated pulse pressure is found in children with hyperthyroidism.

Low blood pressures are noted in children with cardiac failure and in children in a state of shock from causes such as heat exhaustion, circulatory collapse, blood loss, and adrenal insufficiency. Low blood pressure due to adrenal insufficiency is seen in newborns with trauma in the adrenal areas, in children with meningococcemia and occasionally other septicemias, and in children with chronic disease states or malnutrition. Low blood pressure in the arms occurs with Takayasu's disease.

Orthostatic hypotension, a decrease in blood pressure of 15 mm and/or an increase in pulse rate of 15/min, occurs with a 20% loss of blood volume or some reflex vasodilatation or lack of vasoconstriction on assuming an upright posture.

SKINFOLD MEASUREMENT

Place your thumb and forefinger of one hand just far enough apart so that a full fold of skin and subcutaneous tissue can be pinched up firmly from the underlying tissue. Do not pick up muscle. Apply skinfold calipers just beneath your fingers. Calipers should apply a constant pressure of about 10 g/mm^2. Make measurements at the back of the upper arms over the triceps midway between the elbow and tip of the acromial process. Measure mid-upper arm circumference with a flexible tape. Measurements of skinfold help in identifying obesity; those of circumference help in identifying and following malnutrition. Representative values are shown in Table 2-2.

3

GENERAL APPEARANCE, SKIN, AND LYMPH NODES

THE GENERAL APPEARANCE of a child may reveal much more than subtle physical findings. On first seeing the child, sit down and slowly observe the child. Does the child look well or ill? Does the child appear comfortable or uncomfortable? If uncomfortable, in what way? Is the breathing easy or difficult? Is the child in any type of physical or emotional distress? Is the appearance alert or lethargic? Is the child clean or dirty? Is the attitude cooperative or belligerent? Does the child have any gross abnormalities or anomalies? Is the child fat or thin or tall or short? Does the body look malnourished? Is the child apprehensive, and if so, is this due to new surroundings, to the parents, to the examiner, or to the disease? Is the child interested in the new instruments presented by the physician? Does the child obey the mother and the doctor or fight them? If the child obeys, is this because of fear? Is the child excited or calm? Does the child twitch and fidget? In essence, is the child similar to peers or different, and if different, in what way?

A statement of the child's general features should describe the facies (facial expression and appearance) and use terms such as chronically ill, alert, comatose, delirious, lethargic, dull, bright, responsive, hostile, and cooperative. These descriptive terms should start you on the road to proper diagnosis. Dirt, feces, or other signs of neglect alert you to possible child abuse. Also note the interaction between the patient and the parents during the entire examination. Pediatricians are fortunate because their patients, unlike adults, rarely dissimulate. Regardless of what the mother says about the patient, experienced pediatricians know that a child who does not look ill is usually not acutely ill and that a child who looks ill is usually acutely or chronically ill.

During the course of each examination, the child should be completely undressed. In the infant, having the mother completely undress the child before the examination is the easiest method. In the older child, respect shyness and any reticence and examine the patient by removing and replacing articles of clothing.

If the patient is acutely ill, try to determine the system involved and the degree of distress. For example, flaring nostrils point to the respiratory or cardiac systems, and delirium, coma, or convulsions indicate a problem in the central nervous system. Note the nature of the cry of the child. A strong, loud cry may indicate that the child is in pain, is frightened, or simply wishes to cry. Even a strong cry is helpful in diagnosis because it usually indicates that the child is not weak or debilitated. In contrast, a weak cry may indicate that the child is weak, debilitated, or gravely ill. A screeching, high-pitched cry may indicate that the child has increased intracranial pressure or other central nervous system lesions. A hoarse, low-pitched cry in infants may be normal or may occur in children with laryngeal abnormalities, tetany, or cretinism.

Normal newborns may be asleep or crying, but older children are responsive during examinations. The child who is smiling, chattering, and laughing is usually well or only moderately ill. The child who cries constantly may be more seriously ill.

A child who lies quietly with few movements and stares into space may be gravely ill or may have been abused. A child with paradoxical hyperirritability may lie quietly on the examining table only to scream when picked up by the mother. This is a valuable sign, since most children are calmed when picked up, and may indicate a serious disturbance in the central nervous system (particularly meningitis), pain in motion (which occurs with scurvy, fracture, cortical hyperostosis, and acrodynia), or a serious disturbance in response to painful stimuli.

A child with acute illness may have parched skin and tongue, sunken, dry eyes, a weak cry, and an exhausted and lethargic behavior. This appearance may also be seen in children with dehydration or acute or chronic malnutrition. The eyes may appear bright and apprehensive in patients with febrile states.

An appearance that indicates pain is easily recognized, with the child wincing, crying, doubling up, rubbing the hand over the painful part, and displaying general fretfulness and other signs of discomfort. The cause of the pain must be determined. This type of painful facies may be modified in a few disease states. For example, with peritonitis the child lies ominously still, the nares flare, and respiration is entirely thoracic and very shallow. With intussusception the child lies very still one moment and claws, twists, and screams in the next moment. Watch the face of the child for apprehension as you examine other parts of the body. Palpation over a tender abdomen elicits a grimace in the stoic as the child says, "It doesn't hurt." A grimace or changing cry as you palpate over the bladder or in the costovertebral angle may be a real sign of renal disease.

The dyspneic child is characterized by very rapid respiration, flaring of the nares, and perhaps some cyanosis about the lips. The child may be irritable and hyperactive, perhaps apprehensive, and appear to be fighting for air. With carbon dioxide retention, confusion, stupor, and finally shock may be added to these signs.

The facies of a child with nasal obstruction is characterized by mouth breathing, an open mouth, narrow pinched nose, high palate, dull appearance, and nasal voice and may be accompanied by a sunken sternum. This type of facies with swelling over the cheeks may occur in children with hypertrophied adenoids or chronic sinusitis.

The facies of a mentally delayed child is sometimes diagnostic. The eyes are dull, the face is blank, and the child is unresponsive. An excellent characterization of this is given by James Thurber (Thurber, 1953, p. 37) in his description of the housewife who has the radio on all day having what he describes as the "Network Look": ". . . an adenoidal dropping open of the mouth and a vacancy in the eyes, as if perception had just moved out of the mind." Mental delay in children may be due to hereditary factors, maternal infections (especially in the first trimester of pregnancy), congenital anomalies of the brain, or degenerative neurologic disorders. It is commonly due to cerebral injury or sequelae of infections, and it is frequently accompanied by other signs of cerebral palsy. However, mental delay must not be assumed in all children with a dull expression. Children who are deaf or blind or who have specific language difficulties and children with prolonged illness or psychologic difficulties may have a similar facies, easily mistaken for mental deficiency.

Note the *position* the child assumes during the examination. Abnormal, resistant, or persistent positioning may be caused by muscular, neurologic, or emotional disorders. For example, the child with torticollis or cerebellar disease may lean the head toward the affected side; the child with appendicitis or other painful intraabdominal conditions may lie on the affected side with the leg of that side flexed at the hip and knee; and the child with unilateral labyrinthitis may insist on lying only on the affected side.

Likewise, voluntary or involuntary *movement* or lack of movement may direct attention to a particular system. For example, a brain-injured child with spastic paresis may keep the arm flexed at the elbow, and the wrist and fingers may be held stiffly in flexion. With extensive cerebral involvement the child may be entirely in extensor spasticity; with cerebellar involvement the child may be ataxic; and with basal ganglia involvement the child may be athetoid and grimacing.

Estimate the state of nutrition. Acute malnutrition manifests as loss of weight and skin turgor. Chronic malnutrition may be indicated by poor weight, bony prominences, protuberant abdomen, flat buttocks, prominent sucking pads in the cheeks, muscle wasting, poor muscle tone, and slow response to stimuli.

Overnutrition is recognized as obesity and unusual weight gain. (Causes of weight loss and gain were discussed in Chapter 2.)

Development is noted. The patient's response to you and the surroundings using speech, action, and crying should be noted, and you should make a rapid estimate of mental development. Gross deviations from the normal can be seen at a glance if the child appears dull or does not respond. Gross physical development for the age is estimated and confirmed by direct measurement.

Speech is one of the developmental signs least subject to motor difficulty and should be noted in the very young child. A 3-month-old infant may "coo" and a 7-month-old infant may say "ma-ma" and "da-da." A few more words are added at 1 year of age, and short sentences are made at 2 years of age. The 3-year-old child, even if not frightened, may stutter or stammer (see Appendix C). Failure to develop speech may be due to motor incoordination of the speech muscles but is commonly due to a lack of desire to speak because of adequate communication by other means. These children respond to simple commands readily. Other causes of failure to speak include lack of stimulus by parents or environment, deafness, mental retardation, histidinemia, or psychologic disturbances. Severe dysarthria is a sign of spastic quadriplegia.

You can keep a convenient record of development by using the Denver Developmental Screening Test (Appendix II). Markedly advanced motor signs such as early rolling over, early head control with poor feeding, and decreased spontaneous muscle movements suggest spastic cerebral palsy.

ODOR

Some infants and children will have distinct body *odors*. A few of these odors are associated with diseases (Table 3-1).

SKIN

Although observation of the skin is essential in dermatologic diagnosis, palpation of skin lesions should not be neglected. The skin may be exam-

TABLE 3-1
Odors of patient or urine

Odor	Disease
Musty or "mousy"	Phenylketonuria, diphtheria
Maple syrup	Maple syrup urine disease
Sweaty sock	Isovaleric or glutaric II acidemia
Brewery, fishy	Methionine metabolism, oasthouse
Garlic	Arsenic, thallium, parathion, or phosporous poisoning
Bitter almond	Cyanide poisoning
"Tom-cat" urine	3-methylcrotonyl CoA carboxylase (biotin) deficiency
Onion	Selenium poisoning
Acetone	Isopropyl alcohol, methanol poisoning, acidosis
Wintergreen	Methyl salicylate poisoning
Violets	Turpentine poisoning
Pear	Chloral hydrate poisoning
Shoe polish	Nitrobenzene poisoning
Coal gas	Carbon monoxide poisoning
Cabbage	Tyrosinosis
Stench	Foreign body in nose, vagina, ear
Fish (spoiled)	Trimethylaminuria
Fish	Kidney failure
Fresh brown bread	Typhoid

ined as a whole or as each underlying part is examined. Regardless of the method adopted, note the condition of the skin of the entire body at each examination. If skin lesions are found, note their distribution, *color,* and character.

Normal pigmentation is caused by melanin in the skin; depigmented areas are termed *vitiligo.* Small depigmented patches may be caused by tinea versicolor, pityriasis alba or rosea, or dermatophytosis. When they are accompanied by structural or developmental defects, chromosome abnormalities may be present. Unpigmented streaks covering large areas of the body may represent hypomelanosis of Ito, frequently associated with central nervous system abnormalities. In children, vitiligo in small patches shaped like a leaf may be the first sign of tuberous sclerosis or other neuroectodermal disease. Generalized lack of pigmentation occurs in albinism, an inborn error of tyrosine metabolism, and the Chédiak-Steinbrinck-Higashi syndrome.

Localized areas of increased pigmentation (nevi) are common. Note size, color, and presence of hair. Various shades of red nevi are usually of vascular origin *(hemangiomas)*. Small vascular nevi with small radiating vessels caused by capillary dilation may be easily compressed. Because of their appearance, they are called *spider nevi* or *spider angiomas*. A few may be present in normal children if on the arms or hands or high on the face. These nevi are larger and more common on the trunk in cirrhosis or hepatitis.

Port-wine stains are pink to purple with irregular borders. Where they involve the trigeminal nerve, they may cause eye and brain abnormalities (Sturge-Weber syndrome). When associated with the venous system, they cause hypertrophy of the limb (Klippel-Trenaunay-Weber syndrome). Multiple hemangiomas may cause skeletal abnormalities (Maffuci's syndrome or Gorham's disease); others cause intestinal bleeding (blue rubber bleb syndrome). Any hemangioma can be associated with petechiae or bleeding because of trapping of platelets (Kasabach-Merritt syndrome).

Yellow, brown, or black nevi are usually local melanin deposits. Nevi over the lower spine may overlie spina bifida occulta or tethering of the cord. Large coarse nevi may represent the epidermal nevus syndrome, which is associated with congenital anomalies. Linear or circular sebaceous or waxy nevi and giant pigmented nevi over the buttocks may become malignant.

Multiple small pigmented spots are termed *freckles*. Multiple freckles in the axillary region are common in patients with neurofibromatosis.

Increased dark pigmentation, especially over the exposed areas, is most frequently due to sun or windburn. Occasionally, increased pigmentation may be due to hypothyroidism, Addison's disease, hemosiderosis, lupus erythematosus, argyria, pellagra, or other deficiency states. A pellagralike symmetric browning of the dorsal aspects of the hands on exposure to sunlight may be associated with cerebellar ataxia in Hartnup syndrome, a metabolic defect. *Photosensitivity* is also characteristic of errors in porphyrin metabolism.

Light-brown asymmetric pigmented areas are seen in children with polyostotic fibrous dysplasia. Darker patches (*café au lait* spots) are seen in patients with neurofibromatosis and are a diagnostic sign of the disorder in children under 5 years of age, especially if more than five are seen and they are more than 1 cm in length. Another sign of neurofibromatosis is fibromas along the course of a nerve.

Large, flat, black or blue-black areas are frequently seen over the sacrum and buttocks. They are termed *mongolian spots* and have no pathologic significance. Bluish-black, soft, verrucous symmetric areas of the axillae, neck, and knuckles are characteristic of acanthosis nigricans and are sometimes associated with malignancies, genetic abnormalities, drug use, and endocrine diseases.

Look for *cyanosis* and jaundice. Cyanosis is a bluish discoloration of a normally pink area and is most easily detected in the nail beds or the mucous membranes of the mouth. It occurs when a minimum of 5 g/dl reduced hemoglobin is present, regardless of the total hemoglobin. Thus, cyanosis develops less easily in an anemic child, more easily in a child with polycythemia, and not at all in a child with an anemia with hemoglobin content of less than 5 g/dl. Visible cyanosis is not a good estimate of the degree of oxygen unsaturation except when the total amount of hemoglobin is between 80% and 100%.

Central cyanosis is always a cause for concern because of its association with pulmonary, cardiovascular, central nervous system, and hematologic disorders (see box). To recognize central cyanosis, do not look at nail beds or around the mouth. Look at the tongue. With peripheral cyanosis, the tongue is pink; with central cyanosis, the tongue is blue. Peripheral cyanosis is caused by excessive removal of oxygen from blood at the tissue level and is usually caused by slowing of blood through the capillary bed because of hypothermia, local venous obstruction, vasomotor instability, and occasionally shock with sepsis or congestive heart failure.

Other causes of cyanosis include obstruction of the respiratory tract, prolonged crying, temper tantrums with breath-holding, convulsive

---

CENTRAL CYANOSIS

Pulmonary disease

Atelectasis
Pneumonia
Cystic fibrosis

Cyanotic congenital heart disease

Transposition
Tetralogy of Fallot
Tricuspid atresia
Anomalous venous return
Truncus
Pulmonary atresia
Congestive heart failure

states, acrocyanosis, and shock. Cyanosis is seen with as little as 1 to 2 g/dl abnormal hemoglobin from poisoning, such as in methemoglobinemia and sulfhemoglobinemia.

Compare the upper and lower extremities with respect to cyanosis. The lower extremities may be more cyanotic than the upper in patients with infantile coarctation of the aorta or in patients with pulmonary hypertension with patent ductus arteriosus. The lower extremities may be less cyanotic than the upper extremities in children with transposition of the great vessels with patent ductus. Acrocyanosis not caused by heart or lung disease occurs with vasospasm (Raynaud's phenomenon); a blue discoloration of the feet of unknown cause occurs in children with Kawasaki disease.

Veins are normally seen through the thin skin of many children. Distended veins in the arms and legs are usually due to dependent position. Dilated veins elsewhere may be due to cardiac decompensation or local venous obstruction and are also seen in cyanotic children. *Collateral arterial circulation* is rarely seen in children.

Determine *direction of blood flow* if fistula, collateral circulation, or obstruction is suspected. First, empty the vessel by placing two fingers together and then pushing one finger along the course of the vessel for 1 to 2 inches. If the vessel fills before pressure is released, collateral circulation is present. Then release pressure of one finger. If the vessel fills after release of pressure, blood flow is in the direction from pressure release toward the area where pressure is still applied. If the vessel does not fill, replace the first finger, release the second, and similarly observe to indicate direction of blood flow. If the vessel still does not fill, poor circulation in the area is suggested.

The area over a vein may be tender with infection in the vein *(thrombophlebitis)*. When thrombophlebitis becomes extensive and causes obstruction to blood flow, the veins may become tortuous, dilated, and easily palpable. Phlebitis of the deep veins of the legs can be elicited by forcibly flexing the foot and noting pain in the calf (Homans' sign). In children, phlebitis usually results from infection spreading from an area near the vein or from embolism or thrombosis.

Jaundice can be various shades of yellow or green and is best seen by looking at the scleras, the skin, or the mucous membranes in daylight; it may be missed entirely in artificial light. It occurs in the newborn when the total serum bilirubin is more than 5 mg/dl, and it is seen in the older child when the total bilirubin is more than 2 mg/dl. It is caused by cellular or obstructive liver disease or hemolysis. In addition to those seen in the newborn period, common causes of jaundice include any hemolytic anemia, many types of poisons, viral hepatitis, infectious mononucleosis, biliary stenosis, atresia or obstruction, leptospirosis, and choledochal cyst. Jaundice may also appear with infections anywhere in the body, especially pneumonia and congenital syphilis. Jaundice is seen with cholestasis, especially with prolonged parenteral alimentation, and is rarely caused by bile duct stones in childhood, although these sometimes appear after episodes of hemolysis.

A pale, yellow–orange tint of the skin may be due to carotenemia and is most prominent over the palms, soles, and nasolabial folds. Carotenemia is due to excess carotene ingestion but may be an early sign of hypothyroidism. It occasionally occurs in diabetic children. A peculiar yellowness to the skin unrelated to jaundice is seen in children with severe hemolytic anemias.

Note *pallor* or paleness. In darkly pigmented children, it is most easily detected in the nail beds, conjunctivas, oral mucosa, or tongue, which are normally reddish-pink. Pallor should never be considered an accurate estimate of hemoglobin concentration. It is usually a normal complexion characteristic or a sign of indoor living, but it may indicate anemia, chronic disease, edema, or shock. *Plethora,* due to polycythemia, is usually not easily detected in children.

Generalized *erythematous* rashes are common in children with the common viral diseases such as measles, German measles, roseola, bacterial diseases (for example, scarlet fever), toxic shock, drug reactions, toxic epidermal necrolysis, staphylococcal scalded skin syndrome, and Kawasaki disease. Erythematous lesions of varying types appearing simultaneously, with peripheral spreading and central clearing, are characteristic of erythema multiforme. Red patches that expand centrifugally are erythema chronicum migrans, characteristic of Lyme disease. If these lesions are 2 to 4 cm in diameter, painful, tender, and nodular (especially along the shins), they are erythema nodosum. The lesions may be skin manifestations of systemic diseases (see box). Erythema nodosum is more common in girls, particularly at puberty, than in boys. Similar single lesions on the hands, feet, knees, or buttocks, usually making a raised circle with normal skin inside and outside the erythematous area, may be characteristic of granuloma annulare, which may be due to sensitivity to penicillin or other agents. Nontender erythematous patches on the palms and soles (Janeway lesions) occur in children with acute bacterial endocarditis. Serpiginous erythematous "lines" suggest cutaneous larva migrans.

A fleeting, purplish erythematous rash lasting a few minutes to a few hours and recurring at short intervals may be seen in children with rheumatoid arthritis. Erythema that is *annular* or circinate, 1 to 2 cm in diam-

---

CAUSES OF ERYTHEMA NODOSUM

Systemic

Rheumatic fever
Streptococcosis
Tuberculosis
Sarcoid
Crohn's disease
Behçet's syndrome
Rheumatoid arthritis
Stevens-Johnson syndrome
Lupus erythematosus
Vasculitis

Drugs

Sulfonamides
Oral contraceptives
Aspartame
Bromides
Iodides

Other Infections

Leprosy
Salmonellosis
Yersiniosis
Chlamydiae
Cat-scratch fever
Fungal

---

eter, serpiginous, and flat with erythematous margins surrounding intact skin over the arms, trunk, and legs but not on the face is erythema marginatum (annulare). It is characteristic of rheumatic fever. The rash may change from hour to hour.

Localized, painful, hot, erythematous, indurated areas with raised borders are characteristic of erysipelas. Erysipelas is usually caused by streptococcal infection of the skin and is accompanied by high fever. Localized, painful, hot, erythematous, indurated areas lacking the raised borders are characteristic of cellulitis. A blue discoloration in the center, particularly in children under 3 years of age, frequently indicates infection due to *Haemophilus influenzae*. Similar-appearing lesions, particularly around the face, occur with cold injury and frostbite (cold panniculitis). Cellulitis is due to infection in the subcutaneous tissues and may overlie areas of osteomyelitis in the bone or thrombophlebitis in children. Erythematous lines following the course of the lymphatics are inflamed superficial lymph vessels (lymphangitis).

The most common erythematous eruptions, however, are of varying extent and may be due to almost any type of irritation. In the diaper area, erythema is an early form of diaper rash—a type of contact dermatitis—and occurs with Kawasaki disease. Wind, sun, wool, or clothing may cause erythema of the face or other exposed parts. Many other irritants are equally culpable. Excoriation of the convex surfaces of the buttocks is usually due to chafing or excessive moisture. The region around the anus is usually excoriated after loose stools, whereas excoriation around the mucocutaneous area may be due to congenital syphilis. Excoriation of opposing surfaces, especially in the creases of the neck or axillae, is intertrigo and may be due to seborrheic dermatitis or moisture with maceration of the skin with constant irritation. The excoriations are red and scaly and sharply outlined with monilia infection.

Diffuse redness of the hands and feet, especially if accompanied by severe pain, suggests the diagnosis of acrodynia, though boric acid poisoning may be similar. Intermittent pallor or cyanosis of the fingers and toes may be an early sign of Raynaud's phenomenon. This condition is usually painless, may be aggravated by cold or emotion, and is due to arteriolar spasm with sympathetic nervous system overactivity. Faint erythematous streaks, especially near sites of infection or injury, indicate lymphangitis. Bright confluent erythema of the cheeks, as if the face had been slapped, with a warm nontender skin that blanches on pressure and fades in 1 to 4 days is seen in children with fifth disease (erythema infectiosum) caused by parvovirus. Intense facial redness with pruritis is seen with rifampin toxicity.

Discrete nonraised lesions are termed *macules*. The rapid appearance of many macules is characteristic of the exanthemata: measles, German measles, scarlet fever, roseola infantum, and typhoid fever. Distinguishing these from drug rashes is sometimes difficult, especially when the macules are caused by penicillin or atropine. Similar eruptions may be seen in children with rickettsial diseases or infectious mononucleosis and other viral diseases, particularly the echovirus and coxsackievirus groups and human immunodeficiency virus. Similar eruptions are seen in fourth disease (Dukes' disease or mild scarlatina) and in erythema infectiosum. A German-measles like rash was formerly seen 7 to 10 days after smallpox vaccination.

Firm skin and subcutaneous elevations with discoloration are *papules*. Papules may occur with any of the exanthemata following the macular stage and may also occur following any condition causing the appearance of macules. Small gray or white papules are seen in sarcoid. Red, circular, nonhemorrhagic areas that are 1 to 2 cm in diameter over the chest, thighs, or elsewhere with scratch marks may be due to ringworm. A large, purplish, maculopapular, scaly, oval area surrounded by smaller, similar lesions is found in pityriasis rosea. Sharply raised, red, scaly areas over the elbows and knees are characteristic of psoriasis. Erythematous papules over the finger joints suggest dermatomyositis.

Skin elevations containing serous fluid are *vesicles* or blisters. Larger vesicles are termed *blebs* or *bullae*. Vesicular lesions of importance in childhood include chickenpox (the lesions appear in crops); herpes simplex (fever blisters about the mouth); herpes zoster (associated with pain along nerve pathways); insect bites or ivy or other poisons (in exposed areas); molluscum contagiosum (umbilicated vesicles usually over the abdomen or knees); and rickettsialpox (vesicles appear on top of maculopapules). In chickenpox, lesions itch, are in varied stages, and may cover the body, including the axilla and head. In contrast to the other vesicular diseases, pain precedes the appearance of vesicles in herpes zoster.

Bullae may occur with burns and may be a sign of abuse. Bullae may also occur on the palms and soles in children with scarlet fever or congenital syphilis. Rarely, they occur following irritation in children with epidermolysis bullosa, the bullous form of erythema multiforme, or dermatitis herpetiformis. Bullae commonly occur in children with sunburn or ivy or oak poisoning. Small vesicles or bullae are also seen on areas exposed to sunlight in children with recurrent summer eruption (hydroa aestivale). Bullae or other eruptions may appear in children exposed to sunlight who have congenital porphyria.

Bullae at birth followed by zebralike pigmentation are characteristic of incontinentia pigmenti or epidermoloytic hyperkeratosis, which are congenital malformations of the ectoderm. Bullae of the ends of the fingers are seen in children with diarrhea who have acrodermatitis enteropathica and are responsive to zinc. Tender skin with erythema followed by bullae that may rub off (Nikolsky's sign) occurs in children with toxic epidermal necrolysis, a severe disease related to staphylococcal scalded skin syndrome, delayed bullae of the hands and feet in toxic shock syndrome, and Kawasaki disease.

Skin elevations containing purulent fluid are *pustules*. Pustules are usually due to bacterial infection or skin abscesses. Pustules may also be seen after any of the states causing vesicles, in the adolescent with acne, on the finger with herpes (herpetic whitlow), or after poisoning, such as with iodine. Groups of pustules due to staphylococci or streptococci are known as *impetigo*. Deeper infections, termed *ecthyma*, probably start as impetigo. Larger abscesses of the hair follicles or sebaceous glands are *furuncles* or *carbuncles*. Small straight lines or *burrows*, associated with papules, vesicles, or pustules, may be scabies, which are due to the itch mite. These lesions may appear anywhere on the body of the child (in contrast to the more localized distribution on the hands and groin of the adult) and are usually accompanied by signs of itching.

Necrotic areas of the superficial and deep layers of the skin, skin *ulcers,* are common in adults with vascular insufficiency but are rare in children. They occasionally occur on the legs of children with sickle cell anemia. Ulceration occurs before the healing stage of smallpox inoculations, and it may occur following skin destruction by agents such as burns or trauma or following subcutaneous injection of antigens as a result of hypersensitivity.

Petechiae are small, reddish-purple spots in the superficial layers of the skin. They frequently indicate severe systemic disease caused by bacterial emboli or vascular damage, which occurs in meningococcemia, rickettsial diseases, leptospirosis, other overwhelming systemic infections or bacterial endocarditis, disseminated intravascular coagulation, and juvenile rheumatoid arthritis. They are not palpable with inadequate or defective platelets as in thrombocytopenic or nonthrombocytopenic purpura or with increased capillary permeability as in scurvy or leukemia. More frequently, they may be caused by injury or increased capillary pressure as with severe coughing (especially pertussis), allergies in which the cause is unknown, or direct trauma. Paler, red or pink areas that measure 0.5 mm may be petechiae or *rose spots,* characteristic of typhoid fever or other *Salmonella* infections.

Ecchymoses, which are larger evidences of blood under the skin, are usually due to bruising or other injury, but they may be a sign of increased bleeding tendency as in hemophilia, leukemia, or the purpuras. Purple-red bruises are fresh, dark blue or brown are 1 to 4 days old, greenish-yellow bruises are about 5 to 7 days old, and yellow bruises are over a week old and healing. Multiple hematomas may indicate child abuse; if found in the genitalia, sexual abuse may have occurred.

Localized areas of swelling and scratch marks are characteristic of *hives* (urticaria or wheals), papular urticaria, insect bites, scabies, and ivy and sumac poisoning. Localized small swellings or excrescences without scratch marks may be warts. Scratch marks with ulcers, ecchymoses, itching, and other skin lesions may be due to neurodermatitis or may be self-inflicted, factitial dermatitis.

Increased sensitivity to skin pressure manifested by wheals or bright red lines is characteristic of *dermatographia*. This is a common disorder of unknown significance. Especially persistent dermatographia *(tache cérébrale)* is a sign of central nervous system irritation particularly noted in patients with tuberculous meningitis. Dermatographia is easily produced by lightly scratching the skin with your nail and is most easily noted over the back or upper chest. Large wheal formation after stroking may be a sign of generalized mast cell disease (urticaria pigmentosa). In comatose patients, it is common with overdose by depressants.

Subcutaneous nodules may be found occasionally. They are usually due to absorbing or calcifying hematomas, sterile abscesses, or poorly absorbed injections. Nodules over the extensor surfaces of the joints or near the occipital protuberances may aid in the diagnosis of rheumatic fever, rheumatoid arthritis, lupus erythematosus, and granuloma annulare. They may be tender. Red, tender nodules on the fingertips, thumbs, or footpads (Osler nodes) are pathognomonic of subacute bacterial endocarditis. Absence of small, saucerlike areas of subcutaneous tissue with buttonlike nodules under the skin may be due to fat necrosis.

Small yellow or orange plaques *(xanthomas)* may be seen on the skin, particularly about the nasal bridge. They are usually due to local accumulations of fatty substance. Xanthomas may occur as isolated findings, particularly in infancy, or may be a manifestation of any condition causing hyperlipemia, hypercholesterolemia, or hypertriglyceridemia. The reticuloendothelioses may also cause xanthomas. Pigmented or depigmented xanthomalike lesions may be adenoma sebaceum, which is characteristic of tuberous sclerosis.

Cysts may be felt under the skin as superficial masses with fluid. They are usually nontender and may transilluminate light. A cyst over the dorsum of the hand or wrist is most commonly a ganglion—a degenerated cyst of the tendon sheath. Tumors of the skin may be firm or soft and are usually lipomas or fibromas. *Atrophic* areas of the skin may follow injury or the use of insulin by diabetic patients.

Feeling the skin for texture may reveal roughness, as seen in children commonly during the winter, especially after contact with wool or soap. It may occur in children with hyperkeratosis due to vitamin A deficiency, hypothyroidism, and hypoparathyroidism. Rough dry skin, especially over the legs, may be a manifestation of ichthyosis. Thickening of the skin in the flexor folds of the elbows and knees is characteristic of chronic eczema. Hardening and thickening of the skin also occurs in sclerema, scleredema, scleroderma, and dermatomyositis.

Yellow, dirty scaling beginning on the scalp is termed *cradle cap*. Scaling beginning on the scalp and proceeding down the face and body, associated with erythema, is a self-limited form of exfoliative seborrheic dermatitis (Leiner's disease), which appears in the first 3 months of life. Scaling that begins on the cheeks and spreads to the forehead, scalp, posterior of the ears, and down the body is characteristic of infantile eczema. This condition begins about the second month of life and lasts 1 to 2 years. Scaling in the diaper area, sometimes associated with vesiculation and infection, may occur with diaper rash. Scaling of histiocytosis may resemble seborrheic dermatitis. Scaling may occur on almost any area of the body at any age because of contact with a large number of agents (contact dermatitis) or dietary deficiencies of zinc, biotin, selenium, or essential fatty acids. Scaling between the toes, on the feet, or between the fingers may be due to ringworm, epidermophytosis, scabies, or irritants in the shoes or socks. Scaling with plaques or vesicles on the the plantar surface of the foot may occur with psoriasis, allergic contact dermatitis, or juvenile plantar dermatosis. Similar lesions on the sides and ball of the foot suggest dyshidrosis. Scaling, especially of the palms and soles, may occur after any erythematous eruption (particularly scarlet fever) or in infants with congenital syphilis or Kawasaki disease.

Subcutaneous emphysema is felt as a crackling or crepitant sensation under the skin. It is most commonly associated with pneumothorax, pneumomediastinum, and gas gangrene. A similar sensation is obtained if an area over a bone fracture is palpated.

Striae are usually pale white or pink lines occurring in localized areas that are growing rapidly, such as the lower abdomen or thighs of an obese child. They usually occur following overeating or during the growth spurt, but striking purple striae may indicate the presence of Cushing's syndrome. Scars are red or white lines and are evidence of previous injury or operation. They are elevated when keloid formation occurs.

Estimate the degree of sweating. Infants normally begin to sweat after the first month of life. Sweating, especially in the child under 1 year of age, may be profuse and is usually caused by exercise, crying, an overly warm atmosphere, or eating. Profuse sweating in the infant, however, may occasionally be caused by fever, hypoglycemia, hyperthyroidism, congenital heart disease, hypocalcemia, acrodynia, pneumothorax, cystic fibrosis, or fear. A dry skin (anhidrosis) is also normal, but it may be a sign of dehydration, coma, atropine poisoning, hypothyroidism, eczema, or ectodermal dysplasia.

Feel the skin for tissue turgor, elasticity, and edema. Tissue *turgor* is determined by pinching the skin, squeezing out the blood, and watching color change. Slow return of color denotes decreased turgor, a sign of shock. Tissue *elasticity* is best determined by grasping 1 or 2 inches of the patient's skin and subcutaneous tissues over the abdominal wall between the thumb and index finger, squeezing, and allowing the skin to fall back into place (Figure 3-1). It is an estimate of status of hydration and nutrition. Normally, the skin appears smooth and firm and, when grasped as described, quickly falls back into place without residual marks. The skin remains suspended and creased for a few seconds in children with poor elasticity.

Pinch the abdominal skin and estimate the *capillary refill time* (return of color), normally less than 2 seconds. Color returns in 2 to 3 seconds with 50 to 90 ml/kg fluid depletion and in over 3 seconds with greater

Figure 3-1
Subcutaneous turgor or elasticity. It is best demonstrated by grasping
the skin and subcutaneous tissue over the abdomen and allowing it to
fall back into place.

than 100 ml/kg, which is medical shock. This test is inaccurate if heart
failure or hypertonic dehydration is present.

The tissues feel plastic and doughy in children with chronic wasting
disease, peritonitis, or hyperelectrolytemia with dehydration. Little subcutaneous tissue will be felt in malnourished children. The skin will remain suspended and in folds in dehydrated patients. This may not occur
in obese infants. If dehydration is suspected in them, other signs should
be sought. Poor tissue turgor may be apparent in a normal infant a few
days old, especially in premature infants, but they rapidly add fat and
subcutaneous tissue so that turgor is normal by 1 month of age.

The skin normally feels firm, especially over the legs. Calluses occur
frequently on the hands or feet following constant irritation. Thickening
over the knuckles (knuckle pads) may be due to induced vomiting in patients with bulimia nervosa. The skin feels thin and loosely filled in children with chronic diseases, malnutrition, and rickets. It may feel very
soft and flabby in children with flaccid paralyses and in children with
muscle diseases such as myasthenia gravis or amyotonia congenita, as
well as in children with mental retardation. The skin may be soft and
mushy in children with Down syndrome. It may feel hard and thickened

in children with hypothyroidism, whether the condition is congenital or acquired. Other unusual texture is described in Chapter 9.

The skin may be tender to touch. This may indicate that the child is irritable or has central nervous system disease or another systemic illness. It is also tender in children with skin infections, underlying bone or joint infections, or referred pain, particularly from intraabdominal disease. Painful skin over the right lower abdominal wall may signify acute appendicitis. Skin tenderness is also noted in polyneuritis, and children with ruptured spleen display tenderness over the left shoulder. Tenderness may be due to a cryptic foreign body such as a splinter. You should transilluminate (particularly the fingers or toes) to help localize the object.

Impressions in the skin that remain for several seconds following finger pressure occur in patients with pitting *edema*. Edema is the presence of an abnormal amount of extracellular fluid and is caused by an increase of hydrostatic pressure, increased capillary permeability, decreased oncotic pressure, increased retention of sodium or other electrolytes, mechanical obstruction of the lymphatic channels, lymphedema, or decreased excretion of water. Puffy-appearing areas on the body that do not pit or leave marks after pressure or pinching are termed *nonpitting edema*. For example, puffy skin without pitting is noted in the cretin. Scleredema, a rare connective tissue disease, is a firm nonpitting edema affecting face, neck, scalp, conjunctivae, thorax, and occasionally the arms and legs but not the feet.

Edema localized in the eyelids may be the first sign of generalized edema. True, generalized pitting edema is found earliest over the dependent parts, especially the sacrum and ankles. It is seen in children with kidney disease, malnutrition (especially protein deficiency), terminal liver disease, and heart failure of long duration. Adolescent girls show edema before or during menses. Other causes include systemic lupus erythematosus. Edema is occasionally seen without apparent cause on the shins in warm weather. Edema in the first few months of life may be seen in patients with cystic fibrosis. It is also seen in children receiving adrenal hormones and in children with hyperaldosteronism or hyperthyroidism.

Localized edema in the eyelids, face, or lips may be due to allergy (angioneurotic edema), sinusitis, trichiniasis (trichinosis), or insect bites in those areas. Puffiness of the eyelids may also be seen in children after a long sleep or after crying and in children with conjunctivitis, frontal or ethmoid sinusitis, or cavernous sinus thrombosis. Edema of the face and eyelids is common in children with any of the common contagious diseases. Localized edema of the face may occur following severe cough, as in whooping cough or diphtheria. Facial edema also occurs with superior

vena cava obstruction or mass lesions in the chest. In infectious mononucleosis, edema of the lymph nodes obstructs venous or lymphatic drainage. Edema of the legs occurs with thrombophlebitis, deep calf vein
thrombosis, inferior vena cava obstruction, cellulitis, and other lower extremity infections.

The ridges formed by the raised apertures of the sweat glands make
up *dermatoglyphics*. These are best seen with adequate light and magnification or by making finger and hand prints. The otoscope without earpiece
is usually adequate for both light and magnification. The ridges form
arches, loops, and whorls on the fingers; when three lines meet, these are
triradii. The normal child usually has a triradius low on the palm; a triradius with an acute angle in the hypothenar area proximal to the midpalm;
and an assortment of arches, loops, and whorls on the fingertips (Figure
3-2). Usually, approximately seven or eight fingertips will have ulnar
loops and one to three will have whorls. One arch is common in normal
children. Radial loops are rare in the normal. Deviations from these patterns suggest the presence of chromosome abnormalities, early intrauterine infections, gross abnormalities of growth of the extremities, or some
form of congenital heart disease. A triradius distal to the midpalm with
an obtuse angle is suggestive of Down syndrome; arches on all digits suggest trisomy 18 syndrome. Radial loops may occur more commonly in

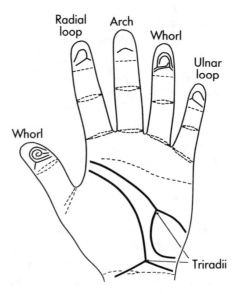

Figure 3-2
Normal hand ridges (dermatoglyphics).

children with XXY anomaly, and large, deep ridges are found in gonadal dysgenesis. Arches on the thumbs are common in children with trisomy 13 syndrome. A single flexion crease on the fifth finger suggests the presence of a chromosome abnormality.

NAILS

The *nails* may be valuable areas for determining special disease states. The nail beds are usually the simplest place for determining cyanosis, pallor, capillary pulsations, and capillary refill time. Vernix in the newborn can usually be found under the nails. Pitting of the nails is seen with fungal diseases of the nails and with psoriasis. Yellow staining of the nails is found in the postmature infant and in the yellow nail syndrome, which is associated with lymphedema and lung disease. Darkening of the nails may be noted in children with porphyria. Nails may be absent in children with ectodermal dysplasia or fetal alcohol syndrome or in infants born of mothers receiving anticonvulsants. Infections around the nails (paronychia) are common in children, especially after desquamating skin lesions. They may be bacterial or fungal infections. Oncolysis may indicate thyroid disease.

Hemorrhage under the nails is usually due to injury, subacute bacterial endocarditis, or other diseases in which petechiae are noted. Telangiectases at the proximal nail folds occur with scleroderma, lupus erythematosus, and dermatomyositis. The nail beds are characteristically more broad than long in children with Down syndrome, pseudohypoparathyroidism, or with congenital malformation syndromes characterized by broad fingers. Spoon-shaped nails with loss of the longitudinal convexity (koilonychia) may be caused by fungal infections, iron deficiency, trauma, or thyroid or intestinal diseases, or they may be congenital. White nails are seen in hypoalbuminemia states, zinc and vitamin B_6 deficiencies, and other types of malnutrition. Transverse white lines in the nails may occur several months after acute Kawasaki disease or other severe illnesses.

Compare the width of thumbnails, first fingernails and great toes. These may be the easiest sites to detect asymmetry or hemiatrophy.

HAIR

Note hair, other than that of the head. Hair is sometimes seen over the shoulders and back of newborn, especially premature infants, but it disappears at about 3 months of age. Children do not usually have hair except for scalp, eyebrows, and eyelashes until near puberty. Long eyebrows and eyelashes are usually familial but occasionally appear in children with chronic or wasting diseases. Heavy facial hair occurs with de Lange and Hurler's syndromes, which are associated with mental delay or endocrine disorders such as virilizing tumors, polycystic ovary syndrome, arrhenoblastoma, and acromegaly. Look for nits or crab lice (a sexually transmitted disease) in these areas.

Figure 3-3
Pubic hair stages in **A,** males and **B,** females. Stage 1 (not shown): preadolescent (no pubic hair). Stage 2: sparse, long, slightly pigmented. Stage 3: darker, coarser, more curled. Stage 4: adult type but smaller area. Stage 5: adult. *(From Tanner JM: Growth at adolescence, Philadelphia, 1962, FA Davis Co.)*

Unusual hairiness elsewhere on the body, especially over the arms and legs, may be a normal variant or familial characteristic but may be found in children with hypothyroidism, vitamin A poisoning, chronic infections, phenytoin or diazoxide use, or hepatic porphyria. Hairiness of the trunk is noted in children with Cushing's syndrome.

Tufts of hair anywhere over the spine and especially over the sacrum may have special significance. Though resembling a nevus, the hair may mark the site of a spina bifida occulta or spina bifida. Nevi may also be hairy.

Pubic hair begins to appear at 8 to 12 years of age (adrenarche), followed by axillary hair about 6 months later and facial hair about 6 months still later in boys. Appearance of hair in these areas indicates normal adrenal and testicular function. Decrease of hair in these areas may be due to hypothyroidism, hypopituitarism, gonadal deficiency, or Addison's disease. Early appearance or increase of hair in these areas may be normal, especially in the obese, but it may suggest stilbestrol, testosterone, anabolic, or adrenal steroid ingestion; adrenal hyperplasia or tumor; acanthosis nigricans; hyperinsulinism; central nervous system lesions; pineal hamartoma in boys; polyostotic fibrous dysplasia; or testicular or ovarian tumors. Pigmented, coarse, curly, or crinkled pubic hair indicates increased hormonal production and is believed to indicate onset of sperm formation in boys (Figure 3-3). Pubic hair without testicular growth suggests hypogonadism.

LYMPH NODES

Lymph nodes are generally examined during the examination of the part of the body in which they are located. Routinely palpate occipital postauricular, anterior and posterior cervical (Figure 3-4), parotid, submaxillary, sublingual, axillary, epitrochlear, and inguinal nodes. Note size, mobility, tenderness, and heat. Shotty, discrete, movable, cool, nontender nodes up to 3 mm in diameter are usually normal in these areas, and in the cervical and inguinal regions, nodes up to 1 cm in diameter are normal up to the age of 12 years.

Nodes that are in the anterior cervical triangle or that enlarge slowly are usually benign. Rapidly growing ones, ones fixed to underlying tissue, or hard, firm, or matted ones are usually malignant.

Absence of lymph nodes occurs in patients with agammaglobulinemia and in some patients with human immunodeficiency syndrome.

Large, warm, soft, tender nodes usually indicate acute infection. Firm, rubbery nontender nodes are more common with leukemia or sar-

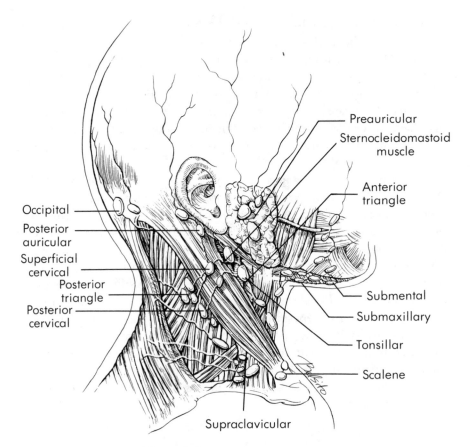

Figure 3-4
Lymph nodes of the head and neck.

coid. Firm nodes that adhere to each other and the skin are found in children with tuberculosis; discrete rubbery nodes are found with Hodgkin's disease, and extremely firm, hard nodes are seen with metastases. Local adenopathy usually indicates local infection but may be a sign of generalized disease. Cervical nodes more than 1 cm in diameter are enlarged. They drain the sinuses, ears, mouth, teeth, and pharynx. The right supraclavicular nodes drain the lung and esophagus; the left supraclavicular nodes drain the lung, stomach, small intestine, kidney, and pancreas; and the axillary nodes drain the breasts, arms, and fingers. For children with inguinal adenopathy, investigate for sexually transmitted diseases or paragenital infections.

Generalized adenopathy is seen with systemic diseases such as bacteremia, streptococcosis, salmonellosis, syphilis, eczema, infectious mononucleosis, toxoplasmosis, histoplasmosis, viral hepatitis, measles, and Kawasaki disease. Generalized adenopathy, with or without tenderness, may be seen in children with leukemia, serum sickness, rheumatoid arthritis, lymphomatosis, Hodgkin's disease, human immunodeficiency syndrome, hyperthyroidism, plague, sarcoid, chronic granulomatous disease, hyper IgE, drug sensitivity, lupus erythematosus, syphilis, or the reticuloendothelial diseases.

A few isolated enlarged nodes may have special significance. Occipital or posterior auricular adenopathy is seen with local scalp infections, external otitis, German measles, pediculosis, varicella and tick bite, and excessive scratching. The preauricular nodes may be enlarged with conjunctivitis (Parinaud's syndrome), styes, or chalazion. The "sentinel" node located near the left clavicle may be the first node enlarged in Hodgkin's disease in children; in adults, this nodal enlargement may indicate gastric cancer. Cervical adenopathy usually accompanies acute infections in or around the mouth or throat, but cool, large, nontender, matted, cervical glands that may suppurate (especially if unilateral) may indicate tuberculosis. Cervical or submandibular lymph node enlargement without other symptoms may herald sinus histiocytosis. When adenopathy occurs near a scratch or bite, cat-scratch or rat-bite fever or tularemia is suggested, as well as disease resulting from tick, flea, or mite bites or local sepsis. The epitrochlear nodes in particular are enlarged in congenital syphilis and cat-scratch disease.

4

HEAD AND NECK

THE HEAD AND neck grow rapidly in the first few years of life and alter the appearance of the child from infancy to childhood and throughout adolescence.

HEAD

By the age of 1 month the infant in a prone position will usually hold the head dorsally. At 3 months of age, the normal infant holds the head steady when held upright by the physician. Failure to hold the head up usually indicates poor motor development. Head nodding may be normal, but it is usually seen in children who are emotionally unstable or mentally retarded or who have spasmus nutans.

Note amount, color, and texture of the *hair*. The newborn infant usually has hair that is fully replaced beginning at about 3 months of age. Lack of hair (alopecia) may be a familial characteristic or a manifestation of ectodermal dysplasia, hyperthyroidism, or progeria. Localized alopecia (alopecia areata) is seen with ringworm of the scalp, other infections of the scalp, and acrodynia, but it is most commonly caused by rubbing of localized areas when the infant lies in one position for a long time. Rarely, alopecia areata is seen in children with localized syphilis or hypervitaminosis A, in neurotic children who pull out the hair, or after severe systemic disease (for example, typhoid fever). Other causes are shown in the box.

Hair is normally smooth with a fine texture. Brittle hair is seen in children with hypothyroidism, hypoparathyroidism, ringworm of the scalp, and arginosuccinicaciduria, a rare inborn error. Fine hair may be seen in any of the states causing alopecia. Fine hair distinguishes hypopituitarism from primary thyroid disease, in which the hair is coarse and brittle. The characteristics of having twisted, irregularly constricted, woolly, or irregularly pigmented hair may each be inherited as an isolated anomaly. Examine the hair for the presence of pediculi or nits.

OTHER CAUSES OF ALOPECIA AREATA

Exposures
X-ray
Caustics

Neoplasms
Lymphoma
Carcinoma
Mycosis fungoides

Skin diseases
Bullous dermatoses
Discoid lupus
Leprosy
Exfoliate dermatoses
Acrodermatitis enteropathica

Other
Collagen diseases (such as scleroderma)
Scalp infections
After antimetabolite or heparin therapy
Arsenic or thallium poisoning

Note the *shape* of the head and face. Marked *asymmetry* of the head is found in children with premature and irregular closure of the sutures. Flattening of part of the head or face occurs in an infant who lies in only one position or who has unusually soft bones. In children with rickets or delayed physical or mental development, the back of the head will be flat. One side of the head and face is also flattened in children with torticollis or may appear flattened in children with facial palsy.

Examine the *scalp*. Special lesions may be noted in the newborn. Scaling and crusting of the scalp, if generalized, are usually due to seborrheic dermatitis or eczema; if localized, they are caused by ringworm of the scalp. Infections of the scalp, which occur frequently, are noted. Lymph nodes and subcutaneous nodules are identified by careful palpation, especially around the occiput.

Palpate the *sutures*. Usually, they are felt as ridges until infants are about 6 months of age. Note abnormal sutures, fractures, and fontanels. The posterior fontanel closes by the second month, the anterior fontanel usually by the end of the second year. A diagram of the top of the head, showing the position of fontanels and palpable structures, is shown in Figure 4-1.

Note the size and shape of the anterior *fontanel* by pressing lightly in the area of the opening. A large fontanel (over 4 to 5 cm in diameter) is found occasionally in normal infants under 6 months of age but may also be diagnostic of chronically increased intracranial pressure, subdural hematoma, rickets, hypothyroidism, and osteogenesis imperfecta.

A tenseness or bulging of the fontanel is best noted if the patient is sitting. The normal fontanel may feel questionably tense in the infant who is supine. Tenseness may be noted in the crying child but only during expiration; this physiologic bulging disappears when the patient relaxes or inspires. Persistent or true bulging or tenseness of the fontanel in the quiet infant in the sitting position usually accompanies an acute increase in intracranial pressure, which occurs with subdural hematoma, lead poisoning, vitamin A poisoning, brain tumor, sinus thrombosis, cardiac failure, meningitis, and encephalitis. Transient bulging of the fontanel has been described in children receiving chlortetracycline, in children with pulmonary diseases, and occasionally in children with roseola or those receiving nalidixic acid or other drugs.

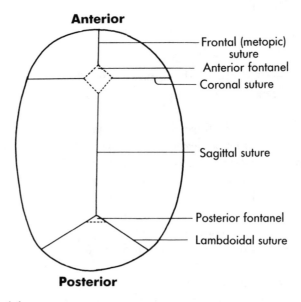

Figure 4-1
Diagram of the top of the head indicating position of fontanels and palpable sutures.

A depressed fontanel is found with dehydration and malnutrition. A small fontanel is usually normal, but it is also an important sign of microcephaly in infants. Occasionally, the fontanel is closed with only fibrous tissue and will feel less firm than the surrounding skull. Fibrous closure should be noted, but physiologically it is comparable to an open fontanel. Bony closure usually occurs 1 to 2 months after fibrous closure. Delayed closure of the fontanel may occur in children with hydrocephalus, rickets, or cretinism. Rarely, delayed closure is due to syphilis or the osteochondrodystrophies.

Slight pulsations of the anterior fontanel occur in normal infants. However, marked pulsations may be a sign of increased intracranial pressure; venous sinus thrombosis; obstruction of the venous return from the head; or increased pulse pressure due to an arteriovenous shunt, patent ductus arteriosus, or excitement. Aortic regurgitation is a rare cause of increased pulse pressure during the age when the fontanel is open.

Measure the circumference of the head as described. Until the child is 2 years of age, the circumference of the head is approximately the same as or slightly larger than that of the chest. Marked disproportions between the head and chest measurements indicate microcephaly, macrocephaly, or hydrocephaly. If the measurements are disproportionate, compare head and chest measurements with standards, since the chest itself may be large or small.

Microcephaly may be due to cerebral dysgenesis alone or to premature closure of the sutures (craniostenosis). Rarely, microcephaly is seen in children with general growth failure.

Hydrocephalus, caused by chronic increase in intracranial pressure, is found by noting the enlarged head, enlarged fontanels, supraorbital bulging, and open sutures. Dilated scalp veins are characteristic of early hydrocephalus. Hydrocephalus is an enlargement of the ventricular systems of the brain and may be due to blocking of the ventricular foramina (noncommunicating), blocking of the subarachnoid pathways (communicating), or rarely failure of the subarachnoid system to absorb cerebrospinal fluid (external). Hydrocephalus is ordinarily apparent at birth or shortly thereafter and is frequently found in children with spina bifida with meningomyelocele. Hydrocephalus starting after birth may be due to a meningeal infection. When it appears in infants at 4 to 9 months of age, congenital syphilis may be the cause.

Bulging of an area of the head occasionally occurs with brain tumors, lacunar defects of the skull, and intracranial masses. Bulging of the frontal areas (bossing) is characteristic of prematurity, rickets, and occasionally congenital syphilis.

Craniotabes is best found by pressing the scalp firmly just behind and above the ears in the temporoparietal or parietooccipital region (Figure 4-2). The elicitation of a ping-pong ball–snapping sensation indicates craniotabes. It represents a softening of the outer table of the skull. Although the infant sometimes cries, no danger is involved if the pressure is not so excessive that the inner table is pressed. Craniotabes is found in premature infants; in some normal children under 6 months of age; in babies who lie constantly on one side of the head; and in children with rickets, syphilis, hypervitaminosis A, and hydrocephalus.

Macewen's sign is one that many examiners like to elicit, but it usually has little significance in childhood. On percussing the skull with one finger, you hear a resonant "cracked-pot" sound. As long as the fontanel is open, this type of sound is physiologic. After closure of the fontanel, the sound indicates increased intracranial pressure or a dilated ventricle.

Percuss the head in children with neurologic disorders in the indirect manner similar to that described for the percussion of the heart. When the head is carefully percussed, you can occasionally elicit dullness near the sagittal sinus. This is a good sign of subdural hematoma.

Tenderness or pain over the occiput may indicate the presence of brain tumor or abscess. Pain over the scalp may accompany cerebral hemorrhage, migraine, trauma, hypertension, vascular neuralgia, and anxiety or depressive states. Press hard over the malar bones for a few

Figure 4-2
Position of hand and fingers (examiner's right hand) to palpate for craniotabes.

seconds and then release. Functional headaches may be improved by this maneuver, but headaches with other causes will not change.

In children over 2 to 3 years of age, percuss the frontal and maxillary *sinuses* in the same manner or by the direct method for tenderness. Tenderness indicates acute sinusitis. Swelling or tenderness on pressure deep in the bony angle above the inner canthus of the eye is characteristic of acute ethmoiditis. It is difficult and generally unnecessary to transilluminate the sinuses in young children. The maxillary and ethnoid sinuses and the mastoids are aerated at 1 to 2 years of age, the frontals and sphenoids after 3 to 7 years of age. The maxillary sinuses can be transilluminated after 2 years of age, the frontals after 7 years of age.

Auscultation over the skull with the bell stethoscope may reveal a swishing sound *(bruit)* of blood flowing through dilated vascular channels. Systolic or continuous bruits may be heard normally in children up to 4 years of age or in children with anemia; after this age, systolic bruits suggest the presence of vascular anomalies, especially arteriovenous aneurysms, or increased intracranial pressure. Similar noise is sometimes heard in children with meningitis. Transmitted cardiac murmurs may sometimes be heard as bruits over the skull. Press over the carotid artery. The bruit disappears if it is *not* due to aneurysm.

Determine direction of blood flow in the scalp veins in children with suspected intracranial abnormalities. You may need to shave the scalp first to determine blood flow, but this procedure occasionally reveals abnormal vascularity or vascular channels indicative of underlying abnormalities. Small ossification defects through which the dura protrudes may occur in the skull. Small defects are termed *lückenschädel,* and large defects are called *encephaloids.* Nerve tissue protrudes in children with encephaloceles. Encephaloceles may be present anywhere in the skull and are sometimes seen near the inner canthus of the eye. On the shaved scalp, note also the presence of dimples, which may be an indication of a dermal sinus or hemangiomas. These are infrequent but sometimes remediable causes of seizures or meningitis. Scalp veins may appear dilated in the very young; they also may indicate the presence of hydrocephalus, tumors, subdural hematoma, or congenital vascular anomaly.

Transilluminate the skull of children suspected of having intracranial lesions. Fit a flashlight with a piece of sponge rubber so that a tight fit is made with the scalp. The room must be quite dark. A sharply delineated area of increased light transmission may be noted over a subdural hygroma. Place a bright light at the occiput of infants suspected of having anencephaly. The light is transmitted through the eyes in anencephalic infants, and you will observe this response as pinkness of the retina.

FACE

Note the *shape* of the face. An easy way to determine *facial paralysis* is to observe the child while crying, whistling, or smiling. The paralyzed or weakened side will remain immobile, and the innervated side will wrinkle. The lips will rise only on the intact side, and the angle of the mouth may droop on the paralyzed side. Wrinkling of the forehead should be noted.

Unilateral paralysis of the face excluding the muscles of the forehead indicates a central facial nerve (supranuclear) weakness and may be seen in children with cerebral palsy or other brain lesions. Unilateral paralysis of the face including the muscles of the forehead and eyelid indicates a peripheral facial nerve lesion and may be due to trauma, otitis media, viral infections, Lyme disease, or other peripheral lesions. Recovery from peripheral facial nerve palsy may occur in the upper portion of the face first, and at this point, it may resemble a supranuclear weakness. Bilateral facial diplegia is a characteristic of Guillian-Barré syndrome. Salivary flow can be measured by putting polyethylene tubes in the submaxillary ducts. Stimulate salivation by placing a slice of lemon on the tongue. Count the drops that occur in 1 minute. If measured in a child with peripheral facial palsy, salivary flow will be at least 40% of normal in those palsies that spontaneously recover.

Paralysis and asymmetry about the mouth only are usually caused by a peripheral trigeminal nerve lesion with weakness of the masseter muscles. Jaw strength can be tested by asking the child to bite on a tongue depressor on each side of the mouth. Beware of malocclusion, which may give the impression of weakness.

Trismus (contracture of the facial muscles) gives the child a sardonic smile (risus sardonicus), which is seen with tetany caused by hypocalcemia, tetanus, or phenothiazine sensitivity and may occur with streptococcal pharyngitis.

Local swellings about the face are usually due to edema. Edema only in the face may be due to any of the causes of generalized edema, as well as allergy and infectious mononucleosis. However, enlargement of the mandible in infants may be due to infantile cortical hyperostosis (Caffey's syndrome) or vitamin A poisoning and may be mistaken for parotitis. Large jaws due to fibrous swelling with upward turning of the eyes is seen in cherubism. A small mandible (micrognathia) is usually a congenital anomaly but may be seen in children with rheumatoid arthritis.

To determine local swelling of the *parotid* glands, sit the child upright, ask the child to look toward the ceiling, and note the swelling below the angle of the jaw. Next, run the flat part of your finger downward from the zygomatic arch. The swollen parotid is then felt. Confirm it by telling the child to lie supine. The parotid falls back like jelly and pushes the pinna of the ear forward. Unilateral or bilateral parotid swelling is usually indicative of mumps, but it may be due to a stone in the parotid duct, an allergy, leukemia, sarcoidosis, or the blowing of balloons or wind instruments. Parotid swelling with lacrimal duct swelling is Mikulicz's syndrome. Parotid swelling due to bacterial infections sometimes occurs in debilitated children. Tumors and cysts occasionally occur in the parotid area in children. Firm swelling of the parotids (parotid sialadenitis) is usually self-limited; it may be caused by animal scratch diseases or may be seen in children who compulsively eat starch. Nontender parotid swelling may precede the onset of diabetes mellitus. Enlargement of the masseter muscles may be mistaken for parotid swelling and occurs in bubble gum addicts or binge eaters, such as bulimic patients.

Palpate the area under the jaw for *glands* or tenderness. Submaxillary glands are felt best by palpating lightly just below the mandible, anterior to the angle of the jaw, or lightly rubbing this area with the fingertips. Sublingual glands are similarly palpated just behind the bony portion of the chin. These glands are ordinarily not palpable, and enlargement or tenderness usually indicates mumps, cystic fibrosis, local infection or infection in the teeth, or rarely, stones in the ducts. Recurrent swelling occurs with Sjögren's syndrome. Unilateral submandibular or submaxillary swelling is more common with atypical mycobacteria, and bilateral swelling is more common with human tubercle bacilli.

Abnormal or unusual facial appearance is also seen in many children with generalized dystrophies, and some of these conditions have characteristic facies. Congenital abnormalities may be seen. Coarse facial features occur in children with mucopolysaccharidoses, hypothyroidism, multiple sulfatase deficiency, I cell disease, Job syndrome, other gangliosidoses, and Coffin-Siris syndrome.

Hypertelorism appears as a large distance between the eyes and occurs with a broadened nasal bridge. It is measured as an increased interpupillary distance and reflects the spacing of the orbits. It is due to overdevelopment of the lesser wing of the sphenoid bone. If the medial canthus is displaced laterally, a similar appearance may exist. This is called *telecanthus*. Both conditions may be normal variants. Hypertelorism with other midfacial anomalies usually occurs in children who are mentally normal. If hypertelorism is extreme or occurs with anomalies other than those of the head and face, the probability of mental retardation is considerable.

Figure 4-3
Measuring interpupillary distance.

Infants with *hypotelorism* and midface anomalies are almost always re-tarded. The normal interpupillary space is approximately 3.5 to 5.5 cm (Figure 4-3). For small eyes, measure the palpebral fissure (the distance between the inner and outer canthus) with a tape. For premature infants, this is normally about 1.5 cm at 32 weeks gestation and increases to about 1.8 cm for term infants. Shortened palpebral fissures are found in infants with fetal alcohol syndrome.

Twitchings of the face are usually due to tics or habit spasms, but they may be caused by muscular exhaustion or fasciculation.

To obtain Chvostek's sign, tap the cheek of the child just below the zygoma with your finger. If the sign is present, that side of the face will grimace. It is difficult to elicit this sign in children under 2 weeks of age or in children who are crying. Chvostek's sign may be present in normal children under 1 month or over 5 years of age. If this sign is present in children between these ages, it indicates hyperirritability and may be found with tetanus, tetany, and hyperventilation.

EYES

A baby's eyes—
Their glance might cast out pain and sin,
Their speech make dumb the wise
By mute glad God-head felt within
A baby's eyes.

Source unknown

The eye is not only the most important sensory organ, but also a key to the brain. A careful examination of the eye of a small child is basically done without the cooperation of the child and is difficult. The infant under 1 year of age may be kept quiet with a bottle, but for children 1 to 4 years of age, you must use other wiles.

Even for a small child, the best examination is done if you use your left hand carefully. Hold the ophthalmoscope in your right hand and keep your left hand far from the patient's eye to attract attention. The natural tendency for physicians is to try to hold the eye open forcibly. This only results in a wet eye that is impossible to hold open, a distraught child, and an overheated examiner. If the child starts to cry when the light approaches the eye, put the light away or let the child play with it and come back to this part of the examination later.

The *sclera* is the white of the eye; the *cornea* is the pigmented area. The clear area of the cornea is round. A small pigmented curtain, (the iris) is normally also round, and by constricting and relaxing, it controls the amount of light that penetrates to the retina and through the pupil. The space inside the iris is designated the *pupil* (Figure 4-4).

Vision may be tested roughly in the very young child by noting the child's interest in a light or bright object and noting the pupillary response to light. A newborn sees only light; by 1 month of age an infant can see smaller objects and by 2 months of age can see rough outlines and follow moving fingers. By 6 months of age the infant should focus for short periods but is farsighted. In an older child, vision can be estimated by the child's interest in brightly colored objects in the room. The eye may be examined by having the child fix, if even for a moment, on some familiar object such as the parent's nose or face. Apparent blindness in a child less than 4 months of age may be due to mental deficiency.

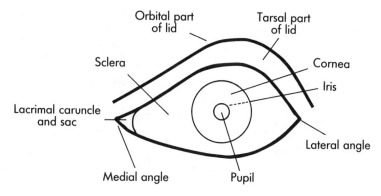

Figure 4-4
The eye.

If more detailed tests of vision are desired, they should be done before proceeding further with the examination of the eye. The infant can respond to light and darkness, and older children will cooperate when tested with an eye chart. The infant may also be tested by rotating a cylinder on which black and white lines are painted. An infant who sees will develop nystagmus as the cylinder is rotated; the blind infant's eyes will remain stationary. This is also a useful test in distinguishing hysterical from organic blindness. Note the child of 1 to 2 years of age while the child picks up different-sized colored objects from the floor. You can test the child of over 2 years of age with a letter E chart by asking the child which way the bars point. Blindness or varying degrees of decreased visual acuity may be due to optic nerve lesions, lesions anywhere in the eye including refractive errors, or cortical atrophy or central nervous system defects. Occasionally, temporary blindness follows head trauma with no sequelae. Unilateral visual defect should focus your attention to lesions that are peripheral to the optic chiasm and in the eye.

If there is any question of a brain lesion, test *visual fields* by confrontation. Hold a piece of cotton in your hand, sit opposite the child, and have the child cover one eye while you close your eye. The child then looks at your open eye. Hold the cotton at arm's length and slowly bring it in, moving it through various planes midway between the child and you toward your eyes. As soon as the cotton is seen, the child will make a sudden movement toward it. This should occur at about the same time you see the cotton. Younger children may be asked to pick up small bright objects.

Vertical defects are termed *vertical hemianopia*. Heteronymous defects are almost always bitemporal, due to pressure on optic fibers at the chiasm. Homonymous defects usually indicate lesions posterior to the chiasm or in the visual cortex; temporal defects usually indicate lesions near the chiasm. Sudden onset of blind spots (scotoma) that enlarge and then resolve may be an early sign of migraine. Central scotoma may be due to pressure on the chiasm or to poisons. Constricted visual fields that are fixed in size, regardless of the distance from the patient, may be caused by hysteria.

The next part of the routine eye examination consists of *observation* of the eye (Figure 4-5). *Blinking* normally occurs bilaterally when a quick movement is made toward the eyes or when one cornea is touched. This is the basis of the corneal reflex. Spasmodic blinking is usually due to habit spasm.

The scleras should be completely white, but they are blue in many normal children because of the normal thinness of the sclera. Blue scleras are found in children with osteogenesis imperfecta, iron deficiency, and

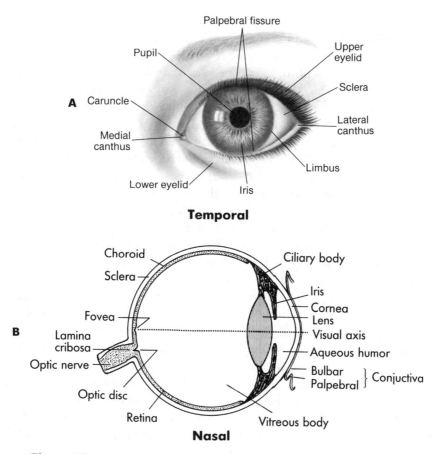

Temporal

Nasal

Figure 4-5
Normal structure of the eye. **A,** Frontal view of eye. **B,** Section through the orbit.

Ehlers-Danlos syndrome. Yellow or mud-colored scleras may be the first sign of clinical jaundice. In carotenemia, the skin is yellow but the scleras are clear. The top of the sclera is visible below the upper eyelid in children with the "setting sun" sign. This sign may be noted in normal premature and sometimes in normal full-term infants. If marked, it is suggestive of hydrocephalus, increased intracranial pressure, or kernicterus.

Note *exophthalmos* or *enophthalmos*. Suspect exophthalmos if the eye appears large or protruding. Exophthalmos due to lid retraction occurs with hyperthyroidism, which is rare in childhood. In children with exophthalmos the distance from the angle of the eye to the front of the cornea is greater than 15 mm. Exophthalmos may be unilateral. The eyes may appear to bulge with congenital glaucoma or, rarely, glaucoma secondary to retrolental fibroplasia. The eyes may be pushed out (proptosis). Retro-orbital or orbital tumors, hemorrhage or metastases, xanthomas of Hand-Schüller-Christian disease, neurofibromatosis, lymphangiomas, hemangiomas, and optic glioma may cause bulging. Orbital abscesses and sinus and cerebral thromboses, which are found especially in debilitated children with bacterial or fungal infections, may also cause bulging.

Suspect enophthalmos if the eye appears sunken or small. Enophthalmos is usually due to cervical sympathetic nerve damage or microphthalmus, but apparent retraction of the eyeballs is observed in children with chronic malnutrition or acute dehydration.

Note the position of the eyes at rest. When the child looks straight ahead, the irises should be between the lids. The iris may appear to be beneath the lower lid with the setting sun sign.

Note *strabismus*. The eyes should be parallel when the child glances in any direction. If there is less parallelism when the eyes move in one direction, suspect muscle paralysis. If the deviation from parallelism is equal when the eyes move in all directions, the squint is nonparalytic or concomitant. An easy method for observing squint is to look at the eyes when the child is looking toward a light about 3 feet away. The reflection of the light should come from approximately the same part of each pupil.

Degree of strabismus can be estimated by degree of deviation of the light reflection from the center of the pupil. Deviation is approximately 15 degrees if the reflection appears at the edge of the pupil, 30 degrees if the reflection is halfway between the edge of the pupil and the limbus (outer edge of the cornea), and 45 degrees if the reflection is at the edge of the limbus.

Another simple test for squint is the cover test. Hold a light about 2 to 3 feet from the eyes, and sit directly in front of the child. Ask the child to focus on the light. Then cover one eye; the opposite eye is noted for motion. This eye is then covered, and the first eye is noted for motion. Motion indicates the presence of strabismus or tropia. Eye dominance can be determined by noting which eye moves a little during the cover test. Resistance to covering one eye more than the other may be an indication of defective central vision in one eye.

Strabismus may be limited to one eye (monocular) or both (alternating). This can be determined by the constancy of the deviation in the cover test. Strabismus may be present only when the patient is tired (intermittent). A test should also be made for strabismus with distant and near objects. Squint may be present for only one of these planes of focus and still be concomitant.

In children with paralytic strabismus the involved eye does not complete the full range of motion. In nonparalytic strabismus each eye can move to all quadrants, but the eyes do not move simultaneously. Paralytic strabismus is usually due to a lesion of the third, fourth, or sixth cranial nerve. Nonparalytic strabismus is usually due to muscle weakness, focusing difficulties, unilateral refractive error, nonfusion, or anatomical differences in the eyes. Always check vision carefully when strabismus is present, especially for equality of vision in both eyes.

Strabismus is frequently present in the newborn, but should be minimal after 6 months of age. Even in the very young, however, fixed strabismus needs a careful ophthalmologic examination to exclude lesions that cause limitation of vision, such as optic atrophy, tumor, and chorioretinitis. Large epicanthal folds partly cover the globe of the eye and may be confused with squint. A unilateral epicanthal fold may be associated with torticollis. Paralytic, usually bilateral, internal strabismus may be an early sign of meningitis, botulism, increased intracranial pressure, and especially tuberculous meningitis. Paralytic strabismus also occurs with retrobulbar pain and otitis in children with petrositis.

Loss of *upward gaze* may be a sign of generalized increased intracranial pressure, pineal tumor, or lesions in the superior colliculi (Parinaud's syndrome). It may be a late sign of kernicterus. Slow movements of the eyes may be observed with any condition causing paresis or paralysis of the eye muscles or with hyperthyroidism. In a comatose patient, deviation of the eye downward and laterally with the pupil dilated suggests cranial nerve dysfunction with tentorial herniation. In these patients, rotate the head quickly. Eyes normally show conjugate movements to the side opposite to the direction of rotation. Absence of this response (doll's eye sign) indicates brain stem or oculomotor nerve dysfunction.

Note *nystagmus* by observing the constant motion of the eyes. Rarely, attempt to induce horizontal nystagmus by having the patient focus on an object from the outer angle of the eye. Record the direction of the fast and slow components of the nystagmus, as well as whether the nystagmus is spontaneous or induced. Circular, elliptical, and latent nystagmus are congenital. Rotatory nystagmus suggests a lesion in the medulla.

In infancy, spontaneous nystagmus may occur in hypothyroidism or may be congenital or of unknown etiology. The infant may be blind and have a peculiar searching type of nystagmus. Nystagmus is characteristic of cerebellar lesions and brain tumors and is also seen in the degenerative neurologic diseases and vestibular diseases. Vestibular nystagmus is always jerky, not pendular. The fast jerks are directed away from the involved ear. It may be seen in children with severe refractive errors. Bilateral, asymmetric nystagmus, pronounced in one eye and hardly discernible in the other, may be a sign of spasmus nutans. Nystagmus present with the eyes shut is congenital or should be considered vestibular in origin. Seesaw nystagmus, in which one eye moves rhythmically up while the other goes down, suggests a lesion near the third ventricle.

Ptosis of the lid may be congenital. It may represent birth injury to the brain or peripheral oculomotor nerve. If it is associated with a sunken eyeball, constricted pupil, anhidrosis, and facial pallor, it is due to cervical sympathetic paralysis (Horner's syndrome). Ptosis may be an early sign of myasthenia gravis, botulism, amyotonia congenita, and myotonic dystrophy and occurs in children with encephalitis or tendon injury to the levator palpebra superior. It may occasionally be noted in children recovering from tetany.

Only slight ptosis results from sympathetic paralysis. Third nerve paralysis results in severe ptosis. Ptosis associated with automatic elevation of the lid during chewing (the jaw-winking or Gunn phenomenon) is a congenital anomaly. Because of weakness of the orbicularis oculi, the palpebral fissures are more widely spaced on the involved side in children with facial palsy.

Other abnormalities of the *eyelids* should be noted. Hemorrhagic discoloration of the lids may be due to injury, neuroblastoma, or any bleeding dyscrasia such as scurvy and leukemia. Distortion of the lid may be due to edema, retrobulbar tumor, or metastases such as neuroblastoma. Extensive infection of the lids may be due to deep abscess formation or osteomyelitis around the sinuses. Fistulas near the lids may be congenital or may be due to chronic infection. Hemangiomas of the lids are very common. Violaceous eyelids may be noted in children with dermatomyositis and scleroderma. Crepitation of the lids (emphysema) is due to air trapping and may follow fracture of the nose or sinuses. Look for distichiasis, a congenital anomaly of the eyelids with double rows of eyelashes or occasional aberrant hairs.

Dark circles under the eyes may be noted. Their significance is uncertain, but they may indicate tiredness, insufficient sleep, or allergy, or they may be a residual of edema in the face. Infraorbital eyelid creases (Morgan's lines) are found in allergic children.

Examine the *conjunctivae* for inflammation, conjunctivitis, hemorrhages, and foreign body. Conjunctivitis alone does not usually produce severe pain—only burning, soreness, or itching. If foreign body is suspected, use a magnifying lens with good lighting. Photophobia may be present with conjunctivitis. The usual causes of redness of the conjunctivae in childhood are bacterial or viral infection, allergy, measles, foreign body, and Kawasaki disease. Conjunctivitis or hyperemia alone is also observed in crying children and in children with eyestrain, emotional upsets, exposure to marijuana smoking, acrodynia, vitamin D poisoning, erythema multiforme, and tridione sensitivity. An early sign of measles, seen occasionally even before Koplik's spots in the mouth, is the appearance of small red transverse lines in the conjunctivae (Stimson's lines).

Conjunctivitis in the newborn is common and may be due to gonorrhea, chemical irritation, or inclusion blenorrhea, which is probably caused by *Chlamydia oculogenitale.* Noting the extent of the conjunctivitis is important. In gonorrheal conjunctivitis or with any acute iritis, the bulbar and palpebral conjunctivae are inflamed; in conjunctivitis due to chemical irritation, the bulbar conjunctiva is usually spared and only the palpebral conjunctiva is inflamed. A dry, wrinkled conjunctiva with foamy, yellow patches (Bitot's spots) occurs in children with vitamin A deficiency. Small comma-shaped vessels in the lower bulbar conjunctivae are characteristic of vascular stasis and sickle cell disease.

Small *hemorrhages* in the conjunctivae may be significant signs of bacterial endocarditis, scurvy, and meningococcemia. They are also seen in the bleeding diseases. They are commonly seen in the normal newborn and in children following cough or trauma.

Pingueculae are small, yellowish, wedge-shaped areas near the cornea. They occasionally occur with the xanthomatoses or Gaucher's disease. *Pterygium,* a wing-shaped white area that may cover the cornea, is an abnormal extension of the conjunctiva.

Styes (hordeolum) are seen usually on the lower lid as tender, reddish-yellow pustules at the root of the hair follicle. Recurrent styes may be a sign of eyestrain, exposure to dust or dirt, general debility, or hay fever, though a stye may be an early sign of diabetes. A nonpainful, yellow swelling of the lid edge (chalazion) is due to inclusion cyst. Scaling of the lid margins (blepharitis) may be due to seborrhea, allergy, or infection.

The cornea should be crystal clear and is best examined with good room illumination or with an open bulb about 2 feet in front of the patient. The cornea is about 10 mm in diameter at birth and 12 mm at adulthood. Any inflammation, ulceration, or opacity is abnormal. The cornea is clear in a child with conjunctivitis.

Note redness of the cornea due to vessel engorgement. If the redness is less near the cornea and increases toward the conjunctiva, superficial inflammation (keratitis) is probably present. If redness is greater near the cornea and fades toward the periphery, deep (ciliary) inflammation (iritis) is present, and the eye is painful.

Opacities in the cornea are usually due to ulcerations. White, Swiss cheeselike superficial membranes at the periphery of the cornea is band keratopathy due to deposition of calcium and is seen in children with hypercalcemia, chronic uveitis, or juvenile rheumatoid arthritis.

Yellow opacities usually indicate active ulcerations; bluish-white opacities are healed ulcerations. Note depth of ulceration. Active ulcerations are usually associated with pain, photophobia, redness of the eye, and a small pupil. If inflammation or opacity is present, suspect foreign body, trauma, or infection. Corneal ulceration may occur with riboflavin deficiency or may be due to herpes.

Pinhead grayish ulcerations with conjunctivitis (phlyctenular conjunctivitis) is a rare painful form of tuberculosis or tuberculin sensitivity. It begins at the corneal-scleral junction and then invades the cornea. Deep ciliary inflammation is especially common in children with interstitial keratitis due to late congenital syphilis. The whole cornea may appear steamy white. Keratoconjunctivitis also occurs with measles and other viral diseases and with rheumatoid arthritis. A gray-green-orange ring around the cornea—the Kayser-Fleischer ring—is seen in hepatolenticular degeneration (Wilson's disease).

Haziness of the cornea is found in children with glaucoma, avitaminosis A, and diseases with hypercholesterolemia. It may also be seen in children with metabolic diseases such as mucopolysaccharidoses and cystinosis, although slitlamp examination is usually necessary to demonstrate crystal formation in the cornea. A large cornea may also be a sign of glaucoma.

Foreign bodies on the cornea or conjunctiva may be detected easily unless they lie over the pupil. If foreign body is suspected, evert the lids and swing the light in different directions while carefully examining the eye. You will observe either the foreign body or its shadow. The lids can be everted by asking the patient to look down. Place an applicator stick just over the edge of the upper eyelid and pull the eyelid forward and upward. If a suspected foreign body or abrasion cannot be located, fluorescein sticks may be placed in the eye. On oblique illumination, the injured area of the cornea will stand out with a greenish fluorescence.

With the light in the same position, evaluate the anterior chamber. Blood or small white spots may be observed. Blood is usually due to injury. White spots may be an early sign of uveitis. Light sensitivity suggests iritis or keratitis.

Note *discharges* from the eye. An infant ordinarily does not have tears before 1 month of age, and the lacrimal duct opens several weeks later. A watery discharge in infancy, usually from one eye, may signify a blocked tear duct. Press on the tear sac, which is just below the inner canthus of the eye. At the same time, slightly evert the lower lid so that you can observe the small opening (punctum). If fluid escapes when you apply pressure, obstruction below the lacrimal sac may exist. Fixed, red, painful swelling and induration in the area of the lacrimal sac indicate abscess formation with blockage (dacryocystitis). Obstruction without infection is usually a congenital anomaly; with infection, it is an acquired disease. A bluish swelling over the lacrimal sac may be a dacryocystocele and should be differentiated from a hemangioma. Tearing with a wet nose, however, may be a sign of infantile glaucoma; with a blocked tear duct, the nose is usually dry.

Watery discharges (epiphora) are also seen with allergy, sinusitis, and styes. Purulent discharges are due to infections. In newborns the pus due to the chemical irritants placed in the eye may easily be confused with gonorrheal ophthalmia. Absence of tears has been noted as a characteristic of children with familial dysautonomia or Sjögren's syndrome.

Compare the pupils for size and shape. They should be round, regular, clear, and equal. Irregularities in the pupil are usually due to congenital malformations. The sudden appearance of an irregular pupil should make you immediately suspect a penetrating foreign body through the cornea. White bands over the pupil may be due to congenitally persistent pupillary membranes. Unequal pupils (anisocoria) are usually congenital, but if they appear suddenly in the presence of equal illumination, they usually indicate acute intracranial disease.

Note *reaction to light* of the pupils. Size and light reaction are controlled by the sympathetic nervous system and the parasympathetics carried by the third cranial nerve. Children's pupils should react to light quickly. Reaction of the pupil in which the light shines is the direct reaction. The reaction of the opposite pupil is the consensual reaction. Absence of consensual reaction on one side occurs with efferent parasympathetic lesion and on both sides with a midbrain lesion. The pupils of newborn infants are constricted until about 3 weeks of age, so light reaction, while always sluggish in an infant with congenital glaucoma, is not a good test of glaucoma in the newborn. Sympathetic nervous stimulation causes dilatation, and parasympathetic nervous stimulation causes constriction. Acute pain or excitement may cause dilatation of pupils.

A fixed, dilated pupil indicates sympathetic stimulation, blindness, or poisoning. It may be caused by pressure on the midbrain due to acute increase in intracranial pressure. It may indicate a homolateral extradural or subdural hematoma, or meningitis. Injury to the ciliary ganglion can result in a dilated pupil that reacts poorly to light but constricts to near accommodation (Adie's pupil). This does not indicate intracranial injury and usually follows injury to the eye. Dilated, unreactive pupils are seen with atropine or deep barbiturate poisoning or anoxia. Coma and acidosis cause dilated pupils. Dilatation of the contralateral pupil on light stimulation of one eye suggests injury to the eye and poor vision of the opposite eye, even in a comatose or uncooperative patient (Marcus Gunn's sign). Pupils that react to accommodation but not to light (Argyll Robertson pupils) indicate a midbrain lesion, such as in those with Lyme disease, viral encephalopathies, and other granulomatous diseases.

The pupils do not react in children whose coma is due to compressing lesions of the brain, but they are usually reactive in comatose children with metabolic disease. The pupils remain dilated in children with partial blindness, but the pupils respond to light in children with cortical blindness. The pupils do not react during a petit mal attack, in contrast to those in children who are staring or daydreaming.

Constricted, unreactive pupils are seen in children with cervical sympathetic palsy (Horner's syndrome); acute iritis; or opiate, light barbiturate, or cholinesterase enzyme poisoning. In neurosyphilis of childhood the pupils remain fixed and small because of parasympathetic injury. Constricted pupils generally indicate that the third nerve impulses are intact.

Hippus is exaggerated rhythmic contraction and dilatation of the pupils. It may be a normal variant but also occurs with central nervous system disease.

Accommodation can be tested even in small children by having them look first at a shiny colored object at a distance and quickly bringing the object toward the eye. The pupil contracts as the object is brought near the eye. This reaction is known as the *convergence reaction*. Various neurologic disorders, including diphtheria, cause loss of the accommodation reflex. Most infants are hyperopic, but occasionally very young infants will play with objects within 2 to 3 inches of their eyes. These infants will probably be myopic when vision becomes fully developed.

The *iris* is usually blue at birth and becomes pigmented within 6 months. Inequality of pigmentation may be a congenital anomaly or may be due to metallic foreign bodies. In Horner's syndrome the involved side remains blue, and the opposite side acquires pigment. Different colored irises (heterochromia) may indicate Waardenburg syndrome. Observe the iris to determine any fluttering, which may occur with subluxation or detachment of the lens. Absence of a part of the iris (coloboma) may be associated with other anomalies or with Wilms' tumor. Adhesions may be seen from the iris toward the lens. These may be congenital, due to persistence of the pupillary membranes, or may occur with chronic iritis, as in rheumatoid arthritis. Black and white spots (Brushfield's spots) in the iris are usually seen in children with Down syndrome. Nodules may be seen in the iris due to tuberculosis, and hypopigmented spots are found in tuberous sclerosis. When a light shines on the iris of patients with albinism, the eye lights up as if a switch were thrown.

Examine the *lens* with direct light from the unshaded bulb. White or gray spots usually indicate opacities (cataracts) in the lens. With cataracts, almost nothing can be seen beyond the white membrane of the lens when the light shines into the eye (see Figure 4-5*B*). Causes of cataracts in newborn infants include rubella in the mother during the first trimester of pregnancy, retinopathy of prematurity, hypoparathyroidism, glaucoma, maternal diabetes mellitus, and maternal thyroid or parathyroid diseases. Cataracts may be associated with metabolic, renal, musculoskeletal, and skin diseases (see box).

CAUSES OF CATARACTS IN INFANTS AND CHILDREN

Metabolic disorders

Galactosemia
Galactokinase deficiency
Diabetes mellitus
Mannosidosis
Hypoparathyroidism
Homocystinuria
Fabry's disease
Refsum's disease
Cerebrotendinous xanthomatosis
Wilson's disease
Glucose 6-phosphatase deficiency

Renal disorders

Lowe's syndrome
Alport's syndrome

Musculoskeletal disorders

Chondrodysplasia punctata
Myotonic dystrophy
Stickler syndrome
Robert's syndrome

Skin disorders

Cockayne's syndrome
Incontinentia pigmenti
Ichthyosis

Craniofacial disorders

Hallermann-Streiff syndrome
Smith-Lemli-Opitz syndrome
Rubinstein-Taybi syndrome
Marshall syndrome
Cerebro-oculo-facial syndromes
Chromosome abnormalities, including
trisomy 21

Central nervous system disorders

Marinesco-Sjögren syndrome

Ocular disorders

Retinoblastoma
Glaucoma
Trauma

Successful *internal examination* of the eye depends on having gained the confidence of the child and having learned to develop a picture image of what you see in a flash. (This same technique is useful in the examination of the pharynx of the child.) Tell the patient that the room will be darkened, that a light will shine in the eyes, but that nothing painful will be done. Eye drops should be avoided but may be necessary. If the child is old enough, ask the child to look at a brightly colored picture across the room. The somewhat younger child can be given a flashlight and asked to turn it on and shine it on the picture across the room.

First, use a +8 to +2 lens to examine the cornea, iris, and lens and then a 0 to −2 lens for examination of the disc and retina. Use your right eye to examine the patient's right eye and your left eye for the patient's left eye. Start about a foot away from the patient's eye, and as you approach the eye, change the ophthalmoscope lenses so that they become less positive. The retina is usually best visible with an 0 to −2 lens in infants and children and is usually seen first as a red area (the red reflex), (Figure 4-6). The details become obvious as you move closer. With this type of illumination, opacities in the cornea, anterior chamber, or lens will usually be seen as black spots against the red reflex of the retina. The anterior chamber is hazy with iritis, shallow with glaucoma, and dark with blood (hyphema).

With direct light, pearly gray, opaque, round areas in the center of the lens are typical of cataracts. Lenticular cataracts are usually lamelar

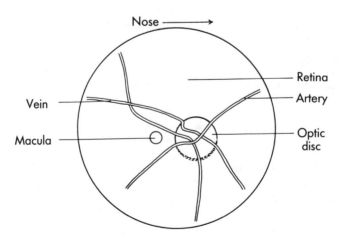

Figure 4-6
Diagram of the retina.

(zonular) in children. The lens may appear clear but out of shape. The posterior eye structures will be seen with difficulty. The lens may be dislocated upward, as in patients with Marfan's syndrome, or downward, as in patients with homocystinuria. Other syndromes with dislocated lenses include Sturge-Weber, Ehlers-Danlos, Crouzon's, Weill-Marchesani, sulfite oxidase deficiency, and mandibulofacial dysostasis.

The appearance of the *red reflex* from the retina is important information. Ordinarily, the fundus will be pink and shiny, but it may be gray in deeply pigmented or in anemic children. The retina becomes gray and loses its shine whenever it becomes avascular. Absence of the red reflex or the appearance of a white-opaque reflex (leukokoria) is noted in children with opacities of the cornea or lens; cataracts; persistent posterior fibrovascular sheath of the lens; retrolental fibroplasia; retinal detachment; or retinoblastoma. Darkly pigmented freckles in the retina occur in children with familial polyposis; a lighter pigment may indicate retinitis pigmentosa, which is accompanied by the complaint of night blindness.

Veins and *arteries* are of almost equal size, or the veins are slightly larger than the arteries. Narrow arteries are seen in the hypertensive diseases, especially nephritis. The vessels are dilated and cyanotic in children with cyanotic heart disease. Venous distention is an early sign of increased intracranial pressure. The veins pulsate normally. Exaggerated pulsations of the arteries, however, may indicate arteriovenous fistula, aortic regurgitation, or other causes of increased pulse pressure. All vessels of the disc are engorged with inflammation of the optic nerve (optic neuritis) and may appear small and thickened with arteritis, as in the collagen diseases.

Fresh *hemorrhages* on the retina in the newborn may indicate trauma or anoxia or may be a cardinal sign of subdural hematoma. In older infants and children, fresh hemorrhages may indicate child abuse. They appear as red spots alone or with a surrounding white haze. These spots are also seen with sinus thrombosis, leukemia, scurvy, bacterial endocarditis, and other bleeding diseases. Multiple, gray, mulberrylike *tubercles* in the retina are seen in children with tuberous sclerosis, tuberculosis, and neurofibromatosis.

Patchy areas of white and red indicate *chorioretinitis*. They may appear in various infections but are characteristic of infection with toxoplasmosis, cytomegalic inclusion disease, syphilis, tuberculosis, and chronic brucellosis. Grayish-brown streaks radiating out from the disc are angioid streaks, seen in pseudoxanthoma elasticum.

The *disc* is most easily found if you relax and gaze from the temporal side of the patient's eye toward the posterior aspects of the eye. The edges of the disc usually have a sharp border around half the circumference and then fade. Blurring indicates increased intracranial pressure. The entire disc may be surrounded by a melanin ring, and this is usually normal. Gray stippling around the optic disc is a sign of lead poisoning. The disc is usually in the same plane as the retina in children. It is usually a little less pink than the surrounding retina. It is very pale in patients with anemia.

The disc may appear large and swollen, the edges may appear blurred, and the retinal vessels may appear to bend down from the disc to the retina in children with papilledema. Such "choked" or bulging discs indicate increased intracranial pressure or optic neuritis. Brain tumors or abscesses, except those originating in the anterior fossa, usually cause papilledema. Pulmonary insufficiency, especially that associated with obesity, may be associated with papilledema (a form of pseudotumor cerebri).

The disc appears white in children with optic neuritis or optic atrophy and may be seen in children with meningitis, encephalitis, other generalized infections, cystic fibrosis (especially in those patients receiving chloramphenicol), many types of poisonings, thiamine deficiency, brain tumors, optic nerve tumors, fibrous dysplasia, congenital syphilis, and neurofibroma. It may precede other signs of multiple sclerosis, or it may be an isolated finding. Unilateral papilledema with contralateral optic atrophy may be due to a frontal lobe tumor (Foster Kennedy's syndrome). If the retina appears opalescent, retinal detachment may be present.

Cupping of the disc in which the vessels appear to dip down from the retina toward the disc may be physiologic or may be exaggerated with glaucoma. A white disc may indicate optic nerve atrophy, which occurs with osteopetrosis causing compression of the nerve and with neurofibroma of the optic nerve. It also occurs following optic neuritis that affects the nerve far back of the eyeball, as with multiple sclerosis or methyl alcohol poisoning, and is congenitally found in children with growth hormone deficiency or diabetes insipidus.

Just to the temporal side of the disc is a small yellow-red area devoid of vessels, the *macula*. Since this is the most light-sensitive area of the eye, the pupil constricts as the macula is approached. In older children, the macula can be visualized if the child is told to look at the ophthalmoscope light. This area appears to be cherry-red in reticuloendothelial diseases such as Tay-Sachs and Niemann-Pick disease and in other cerebromacular degenerative diseases. The macula may be brown and appear fragmented in children with the juvenile form of macular degeneration. Bruit over the eyeball may occur with congenital arteriovenous fistulas in the brain.

Later in the examination, obtain the *corneal reflex* by touching the cornea with a piece of cotton. Both eyes normally shut, since this is painful. Failure to obtain the corneal reflex indicates trigeminal (sensory component) or facial (motor component) nerve injury. Pontine injuries and anesthesia depress this reflex.

In general, complete cooperation is impossible with young children. As the child gets older, devices for obtaining attention should be used. However, with or without cooperation, you should explore these areas of the eye. If you note a defect in any area, refer the patient to an ophthalmologist, who can use other instruments and anesthetics.

EARS

Except for thermolabile children, the most common cause of fever without obvious reason in childhood is ear infection. Examine the ears of all sick children.

Various *anomalies* of the ears occur (Figure 4-7). These are usually obvious deformities of the auricle. Occasionally, a small sinus is present as a hole or pit just in front of the ear, and this may be accompanied by a small swelling just inside the canal; this represents the remnant of the first brachial cleft.

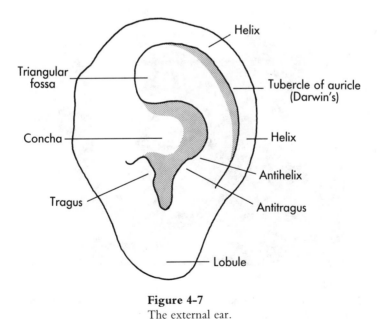

Figure 4-7
The external ear.

Note the *position* of the ears. In infants with Potter's syndrome, the tops of the ears are below the level of the eye and there is congenital absence of the kidneys. Other gross anomalies of the ears may be associated with lesser kidney anomalies.

The auricles frequently appear to stand forward with any mass or swelling behind the ear. Important conditions causing this appearance are mastoiditis, cellulitis, mumps, and postauricular abscesses. Occasionally, enlarged postauricular nodes or external otitis with surrounding cellulitis makes the ears protrude.

Note the nature and odor of discharge from the aural canals. A greenish, foul-smelling discharge occurs with pyocyanic infections. Purulent discharges are seen with any bacterial infection, particularly *Streptococcus pneumoniae* and *Mycobacterium tuberculosis,* but may also occur with fungal infections of the canal wall. Generalized eczema may cause flaking in the ears. Bloody discharge is usually due to scratching, irritation, or injury of the ear canal but may occur with foreign body in the canal or be a cardinal sign of basilar skull fracture.

Next, the otoscope is used (Figure 4-8). First, the otoscope should be halogen illuminated and operating properly with fresh batteries or the light will turn yellow. Second, the largest possible green nylon speculum should be used. The speculum must be cleaned before use and should

Figure 4-8
Using the otoscope. The hand holding the otoscope rests firmly on the patient's head or face.

never enter the canal more than 10 to 15 mm. The only use for the 1- or 2-mm speculum, even in infants, is to cloud the field and hurt the patient. Third, examine the canal before you try to look at the drum to note the presence of a furuncle or vesicle in the outer edge of the canal. If a furuncle is hit with the otoscope, the child will feel pain and the examination will probably end! Fourth, hold the otoscope firmly with one hand, and as the speculum is inserted, rest the hand holding the otoscope firmly on the child's head or face so that any motion by the child will be accompanied by a similar movement of the otoscope. Fifth, placing the speculum just inside the canal of one ear and then the other before attempting to examine the drum is also valuable. This assures the child that the procedure will not hurt. Examining the child's doll first or looking for an elephant in the ear may also reassure the child. Finally, before using the otoscope, remember the direction of the canal. In infants, the canal is directed upward, so the auricle should be pulled down to view the drum. In older children, the canal faces downward and forward, so pull the tip of the auricle up and back for adequate visualization. Pulling the external ear serves another useful purpose. Ordinarily, this movement is painless in children with otitis media and in children without an ear infection, but it is painful in children with a furuncle in the ear or external otitis.

Examination of the ears should be almost painless. Allow the child to play with the otoscope, but at the time of the examination, handle the child firmly. Either the child assures you of cooperation or the mother holds the child so that the head does not move and the hands do not interfere. The child should be placed face down and prone, with the head turned first to one side, then the other. Tell the child that the speculum plays a song but that the child must be very quiet to hear it. After examining the first ear, ask if the song was heard. Then repeat the procedure in the opposite ear.

The *canal* and auricle may be swollen in children with external otitis, as occurs with seborrhea and allergic dermatitis, or in nervous children who frequently place foreign bodies in the canal. Note any tenderness. Tenderness as the speculum is placed in the canal may indicate disease of the canal, such as a furuncle, or disease of the middle ear (otitis media). Vesicles in the canal may be due to viral canal infections or otitis media caused by *Haemophilus influenzae*. If cerumen is present, a large enough speculum frequently allows you to look above or below the wax at the drum. If a small, easily reached foreign body or obstructive wax is present, it is best removed with an ear spoon or wire loop.

Discharges may arise from the canal, external otitis, otitis media with perforation of the drum, or chronic otitis media with mastoiditis. Swimmer's discharge is usually due to gram–negative bacilli. Greenish discharge is usually from external otitis. Mucoid or mucopurulent discharge most often arises from the middle ear. Carefully wipe away discharges with a soft, cotton–tipped applicator. Be careful to blot the discharge so that nothing is pushed against the ear drum, which may be perforated. Do not use cotton–tipped applicators for removing hard wax or foreign bodies.

Rarely, you may resort to the use of an ear syringe to remove adherent wax. First, soften the wax with a detergent. Fit the syringe with a narrow "fistula tip" to provide a thin stream. Fill the syringe with lukewarm water (cover the patient to prevent soaking), and introduce it gently into the tip of the canal, which is then flushed. This procedure is unpleasant and undesirable in examining children because a vestibular response, frequently with vomiting, is induced. It should never be done if a perforation of the drum is suspected or if a foreign body is in the canal.

The normal *drum* (Figure 4-9) is gray–white and translucent or opalescent. The handle of the malleus appears as a small white streak running down and back to the center of the ear and ends at the umbo. At the upper end of the malleus is a small white projection, the short process of the malleus. Below the umbo is a small circle of light, the light reflex. Even in the infant, whose drum is almost horizontal, determine these landmarks. As the child gets older, the drum becomes vertical but points inward. The light reflex becomes cone shaped and sharply outlined, with the apex at the center and the base at the anterior–inferior portion of the drum.

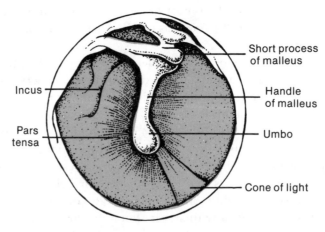

Figure 4-9
Diagram of the tympanic membrane (ear drum).

The most common abnormality of the drum noted on otoscopic examination is slight redness. This may be due to crying or to manipulation. If the drum is slightly to markedly reddened and retracted as noted by the prominence of the malleus and a deeper and sharper outline of the cone of light and if the vessels are prominent, catarrhal otitis media is present. This is usually due to any upper respiratory infection or to obstruction of the eustachian tube. The light reflex may appear less prominent than usual.

In acute suppurative otitis media, the *light reflex* is usually lost, the drum bulges outward and becomes diffusely red, the handle of the malleus is not seen clearly, and hearing is usually decreased. Occasionally with a bulging drum, the light reflex is scattered diffusely over the drum area instead of being lost. Recognize that this reflex is coming from a convex drum, since the handle of the malleus is not seen. Otitis media in the young infant may be due to congenital syphilis in addition to the usual causes of suppuration, such as *H. influenzae,* pneumococci, streptococci, staphylococci, and viruses. Otitis, sometimes with mastoiditis and abducens paralysis of the homolateral eye, occurs with petrositis (Gradenigo's syndrome). Chronic otitis may be due to tuberculosis or other bacterial infections, immune defects, allergy, and histiocytosis. It may also be associated with enlarged adenoids, cleft palate, and mastoiditis. Otitis in the infant may be caused by the infant having been fed frequently with a propped bottle or in the supine position.

Bulging may also be due to nonpurulent fluid. This occurs in children with late catarrhal otitis media or suppurative otitis in which the bacterial infection has resolved but the exudate has not yet been resorbed (serous otitis). Bulging with a bluish discoloration of the drum may be due to a collection of blood in the middle ear and occurs after trauma and sometimes after infection. Blood behind the drum suggests basilar skull fracture.

The drum may be *perforated.* Perforation with pus indicates acute or chronic purulent otitis media. Small perforations may be seen in the drum due to injury, insect bites, or chronic tuberculosis. You may prefer to quantitate the conducting mechanism of the ear by tympanometry, which helps document fluid in the inner ear, drum perforation, and other changes in air and sound conduction.

Myringitis may be indicated if you find varying degrees of redness of the drum, with possibly some loss of the light reflex but without bulging or retraction or evidence of fluid in the middle ear, especially if accompanied by exquisite pain and little hearing loss. Myringitis is a primary inflammation of the drum head without involvement of the middle ear, or it may be an early stage of otitis media.

Occasionally, you will see a small mass (usually gray, red, or yellow) just in front of or behind the drum from which pus oozes. This is a cholesteatoma. A pinpoint perforation may accompany it in the posterior-superior or central portion of the drum.

Note *mobility* of the drum. This requires a tight-fitting otoscope and speculum with a hole through which a puff of air can be introduced with an attached rubber bulb. Another option is to attach a tube to the otoscope, place the other end in your mouth, and blow in and suck out. The light reflex and drum will move. An immovable drum is found in suppurative or serous otitis media. Serous otitis is a condition with conductive hearing loss with a fluidlike secretion in the middle ear. It may be caused by allergies, chronic infections, hypothyroidism, obesity, or anything that contributes to the closure of the eustachian tube. An immovable drum is also found in children with osteopetrosis.

Next, feel and tap the *mastoid* tip of the temporal bone. Note any fluctuation or tenderness; either may indicate mastoiditis. Just behind the mastoid, feel for the postauricular nodes. In children, these are normally about 1 or 2 mm in diameter. Enlarged nodes are characteristic of German measles, nits, or inflammation of the scalp and are usually slightly tender. They are also found in children with measles, roseola, varicella, infectious mononucleosis, leukemia, and tick bites. In this area, you may occasionally feel subcutaneous nodules about 2 to 5 mm in diameter. These nodules are characteristic of active rheumatic fever.

Estimate *hearing*. In small children, make a sharp noise at the child's ear and note a blinking of the eyes. Each ear is tested separately while you stand outside the direct line of vision of the child. In older children, testing by using the whispered voice at a distance of about 8 feet is sufficient. This is best done by asking the child simple questions or whispering a simple command. Nothing is quite so gratifying as diagnosing impaired hearing in a child who was thought to be mentally defective. Many children will tell you that they hear a watch tick when it is held about 6 to 10 inches from the head. You can develop this into a relatively quantitative hearing test by using your watch with a number of normal children and determining how far from the ear the watch can be heard.

Loss of hearing can be conductive, neurosensory, or mixed. Over the age of 3, most mentally normal children are cooperative enough to be tested with a *tuning fork*. If your hearing is normal, press the tip of the vibrating tuning fork against the mastoid process of the child and then of yourself. The number of seconds it is heard by both is compared. If the child hears it for less time than you, this indicates decreased bone conduction, a sign of neurosensory hearing loss. If the child hears it longer, this indicates conductive loss (Schwabach test). Compare air and bone conduction in the patient. First place the fork on the mastoid as before and then about 1 inch from the ear with approximately equal vibratory stimulus. Normally, air conduction is twice as long as bone conduction (Rinne's test). Then place the vibrating fork on the middle of the child's forehead and ask in which ear the sound is heard better. In unilateral conductive deafness, the hearing is better in the unaffected side (Weber's test). In unilateral neurosensory deafness, the hearing is better in the affected ear.

Hearing loss may be due simply to foreign body or cerumen in the canals. Defective hearing may be noted in children with chronic catarrhal otitis media associated with enlarged adenoids or other nasal obstruction, in children who have received dihydrostreptomycin, or in children who have had meningitis, encephalitis, kernicterus, or Hunter's syndrome. Congenital deafness is usually idiopathic, or it may be found in children whose mothers had rubella during the first trimester of pregnancy. Unilateral deafness may follow mumps. Deafness associated with syncope may be due to congenital heart lesions (Jervell and Lange-Nielsen syndrome). Deafness may be associated with hereditary renal disease with hyperprolinemia or with a white forelock and eye abnormalities (Waardenburg syndrome). Pseudodeafness may be seen in psychotic children, especially those with autism, or in children with mental deficiency. More complicated types of deafness should be referred to an otologist. Hyperacute hearing may occur in children with Tay-Sachs disease or tetanus.

Children who have received streptomycin or who have nystagmus or an unsteady gait or dizziness *(vertigo)* should have their *vestibular* function tested. The cold caloric test usually suffices. Seat the patient and inject water of 65° F (18° C) into the ear. Nystagmus should appear within 30 seconds, with the fast movement opposite the injected ear. Fast movement toward the injection suggests central nervous system disease. Repeat in the opposite ear. Nystagmus should persist almost equally (for about 1 to 2 minutes) on each side. Lack of nystagmus suggests lack of labyrinth function or vestibular or brain stem disease. This may be due to streptomycin medication, labyrinthitis, meningitis, or brain tumor, or it may be a sign of benign paroxysmal vertigo. Vertigo with tinnitus and fluctuating hearing loss is characteristic of Ménière's disease. Dizziness with progressive hearing loss and facial or corneal numbness occurs with acoustic neuroma. Acute vertigo with nausea and vomiting followed by dysarthria, dysphagia, or unilateral weakness suggests infarct in the medulla with posterior cerebellar or vertebral artery involvement (Wallenberg's syndrome). Hiccups may accompany the vertigo. Vertigo with nystagmus that occurs after putting air pressure on the drum indicates a fistula, especially with cholesteatoma.

NOSE

Examination of the nose, even superficially, is often neglected. Yet it may hold the key to the proper diagnosis.

Note any unusual *shape* of the nose. Because the lower half of the nasal septum is cartilage, you will rarely see fracture or dislocation of the nose in childhood. Deviation is occasionally seen in the newborn, perhaps due to intrauterine position. The chief cause of flattening of the nose in childhood is cleft palate. With cleft palate the nasal septum is deflected and the nose appears flattened. A saddle-shaped nose is characterized by a low bridge and broad base. This is usually seen as a familial characteristic but also occurs in children with hypertelorism or following perforation of the septum, as in congenital syphilis.

Note *flaring* of the alae nasi. The alae flare with all types of respiratory obstruction or distress but particularly with pneumonia. Flaring of the alae nasi may be seen in children with fevers, acidosis, peritonitis, or any condition or illness causing anoxia.

Next, shine a light up the nose and note the color of the *mucosa*. If you push the tip of the nose upward with the thumb of your left hand and hold the light with your right hand, you can frequently see high into the nose. A speculum is usually not necessary for satisfactory examination of the mucosa or the ostia of the sinuses. If a nasal speculum is desired, use the spring-type rather than the otoscope speculum. By placing the large otoscope speculum in the tip of the nose, you can examine the area to the middle meatus. The nasal speculum is preferably used with a head mirror, but satisfactory examination can be performed with a hand light if the mother holds the baby's head firmly. A red, inflamed mucosa indicates infection, including sinusitis. A pale, boggy mucosa may indicate allergy. A swollen grayish mucosa may indicate chronic rhinitis.

Note the character of secretions. Purulent secretions are common with any nasal infection, even the usual upper respiratory infection in its later stages, or may be an early sign of the contagious diseases, particularly measles, pertussis, and poliomyelitis. Purulent secretions from the ostia above or below the middle turbinates indicate sinusitis; pus in the middle meatus suggests involvement of the maxillary, frontal, or anterior ethmoid sinuses; and pus in the superior meatus suggests involvement of the posterior ethmoid or sphenoid sinuses. Patients with discharge and crusting below or on the edges of the alae nasi, particularly with redness of the surrounding skin, usually have infections with β-hemolytic streptococci. Purulent discharges may also be caused by *H. influenzae* or *S. pneumoniae*. Purulent or bloody secretions in infancy may be a sign of secondary syphilis. When due to syphilis, they may occur in children up to the age of 6 months and are usually associated with excoriations of the upper lip.

Watery nasal secretions may indicate allergy, the common cold, foreign bodies high in the nose, illicit drug use, or rarely, skull fracture or perforated encephalocele. Unilateral purulent secretions suggest foreign body, nasal diphtheria, nasal polyps, and sinusitis.

Note *bleeding points* in the nose. They are most commonly found at the lower anterior tip of the septum. Epistaxis is rare in infancy and may indicate a bleeding dyscrasia if present. The usual cause of epistaxis, hemoptysis, and hematemesis in children is irritation or injury of the nasal mucosa. Epistaxis is especially common in children with allergic rhinitis. Other less common causes of epistaxis include nasal infections (particularly diphtheria); typhoid fever; leukemia; rheumatic fever; foreign body; and congestion due to any cause such as congenital heart disease. Occasionally, epistaxis in childhood is caused by late syphilis, elevated blood pressure due to any cause, or any of the anemias or bleeding diseases. Bleeding after skull injury may be due to local nasal injury or to skull fracture. Rarely, a bleeding telangiectasis is seen in the mucosa and may be the cardinal sign of familial telangiectasia. Epistaxis may be the only physical sign of hereditary hemorrhagic thrombasthenia, one of the bleeding diseases.

Note the child's ability to get air through the nose. Infection, foreign body, vasomotor rhinitis, tumor, polyp, or a badly deviated septum are the usual causes of inability to breathe through the nose. The newborn with bilateral choanal atresia is unable to get air through the nostrils and often appears to be choking. In the older child, large adenoids, even if uninfected, may cause nasal obstruction with a typical adenoid facies. Obstruction with recurrent epistaxis, especially in teenage boys, suggests angiofibroma.

An unusually large nasal airway with dry crusting is occasionally noted. This may be a sign of atrophic rhinitis, which occurs in older children or adults. A malodorous nasal discharge may be present.

In the older child, examine the nasal *septum*. Perforation may be due to injury of the nasal septum, foreign body, syphilis, tuberculosis, or sniffing of illicit drugs. The nasal septum is deflected in children with cleft palate or injury.

Occasionally *polyps* or *tumors* may occlude one nostril or even protrude from the nose. Polyps frequently occur with allergy but may be a manifestation of chronic infection, cystic fibrosis, or generalized polyposis. An encephalocele may protrude through the cribriform plate and appear to be a polyp. If you see a membrane in the nose preceded by bleeding, consider diphtheria until this diagnosis can be eliminated.

Percuss the sinus areas as previously described for evidence of pain. Olfactory nerve tests are generally not done in childhood. Anosmia is a sign of Kallmann's syndrome, zinc deficiency, and chronic nasal infection.

MOUTH AND THROAT

Defer examination of the mouth and throat until the end of the examination in young children. For you to see the posterior pharynx and particularly the epiglottis during gagging, the child must be sitting and cooperative or adequately restrained when the depressor is finally placed far in the mouth. If the mother or an assistant is present, the child can sit on this person's lap. Ask the mother or assistant to hold both the child's wrists with one hand and the forehead with the other (Figure 4-10).

As in the examination of the fundus of the eye, a photographic memory is helpful. In many children, a brief glimpse of the interior of the mouth is all that you will obtain. Giving the child a tongue depressor while the examination is proceeding is usually helpful. Ask the child to

Figure 4-10
Restraint of patient in sitting position to examine posterior pharynx and epiglottis.

open the mouth while the child holds the tongue depressor. Examine the external structures first.

Around the mouth, note *circumoral pallor*. With circumoral pallor the immediate area around the mouth appears white, and the strip just below the nose, the surface of the cheeks, and the lower chin are red. This appearance may occur with any febrile disease, but it is particularly noted in children who have just exercised or who have scarlet or rheumatic fever or hypoglycemia. Even in infants with seborrheic dermatitis and eczema, this pale area usually remains free of lesions, although the remainder of the cheeks may be covered with scales.

Inspect the *lips*. Asymmetry of the mouth with twisting of the lips to one side is found with facial nerve or trigeminal nerve paralysis. Cleft lip, usually on the left side, is a congenital anomaly. Note extent and location of the cleft. Lip pits may appear as isolated deformities or may be associated with other anomalies.

Slight *fissures* of the lips (cheilitis) are seen in children exposed to wind and sun and in children with Kawasaki disease. Rhagades are deep fissures or their resultant scars coming from the nose to the lips and extending outward from the lips. They are characteristic of congenital syphilis. Deep radiating painful fissures from the ends of the lips (cheilosis) are seen in children with numerous nutritional disturbances, particularly riboflavin and other B vitamin, protein, or iron deficiences, or with *Candida* and other infections. Excoriation of the upper lip occurs frequently in young children with simple upper respiratory infections. Painful ulcers on the lips and adjacent tissues are characteristic of erythema multiforme.

Vesicles and pustules appear on the lips in older children, especially following upper respiratory infections. "Cold sores" (herpes simplex) are vesicles on an inflamed base and usually burn or itch. Bacterial infections are detected as ordinary pustules. Retention cysts, usually single, occur on the lip and appear as small protrusions containing clear fluid.

Note the *color* of the lips. The normal pink of white children and gray of black children is replaced by a pale mucosa when anemia is present. Gray cyanosis is seen with most congenital heart lesions, methemoglobinemia, anoxia, and bizarre poisons. Deep-purple lips are seen with severe congenital heart disease. Cherry-red lips are characteristically seen in infants and children with acidosis and are frequently due to aspirin poisoning or diabetes in older children. Cherry-red lips are also seen in patients with carbon monoxide poisoning. With many poisons the lips may appear red although the remainder of the body is pallid. Telangiectases in the lips may herald Rendu–Osler–Weber syndrome (familial telangiectasia).

The lips may be grossly *swollen* due to insect bites, local infection or injury, angioneurotic edema, or massive generalized edema.

Note unusual *odors* from the mouth. The sweetish odor of acetone is common in dehydrated or malnourished children but may indicate diabetic acidosis as in adults. A mouselike odor occurs in children with diphtheria. A peculiar odor similar to that obtained from decaying tissue may occur in children with typhoid fever. An ammoniacal odor occurs in children with uremia. Halitosis (bad breath) occurs in children with many varied states, including poor local hygiene, local or systemic infections, sinusitis, and mouth breathing.

It is useless to ask a child less than 6 or 7 years of age if the throat hurts, since even with acute pharyngitis or tonsillitis, the child usually has no pain. If pain is present in younger children, it more commonly indicates the presence of epiglottitis or laryngitis or occasionally abscess, diphtheria, or scarlatina.

Most patients will open their mouths when asked to do so. Inability of a child to open the mouth is generally only voluntary and not a real inability. Real inability to open the mouth occurs with tetanus (trismus), tetany, infections in the tissues surrounding the mouth, peritonsillar abscess, dislocation of the temporomandibular joint, and occasionally, parotitis. In rheumatic fever or rheumatoid arthritis the swollen temporomandibular joint will sometimes prevent the patient from opening the mouth. Ankylosis of the joint may occur secondary to birth injury to the joint. Temporomandibular joint involvement can frequently be recognized not only by the apparent inability to move the joint, but also by obvious asymmetry of the face. Trismus may also occur in children with infantile Gaucher's disease, brain tumor, or encephalitis, and it is noted frequently in children who receive phenothiazine derivatives.

If the child does not open the mouth after suggestion, tell the child to show the teeth. Most children aged 2½ or older will open the mouth, and the posterior pharynx can be visualized if the child is asked to say "ah" or "eh." If the child declines, place the tongue blade gently between the lips and push the mucosa away from the teeth to obtain an adequate view of the teeth, gums, and mucosa. If mouth lesions are suspected, it is frequently less painful if the tongue blade is moistened before insertion. Examine the throat at this time. Do not restrain patients unless they move. In older children, if you push down first one side of the tongue and then the other, it is sometimes easier to visualize all the mouth and throat. Good lighting, preferably daylight, is necessary for further examination.

It is important, however, to become accustomed to the use of one type of light, either daylight or electric. You are then familiar with the appearance of the structures with this light.

Inspect the *teeth* for number, caries, and type of occlusion. Compare the number of teeth present with the averages for the age (Table 4-1). Occasionally a tooth will be seen in the newborn. Delayed appearance of the deciduous teeth (for example, after 1 year of age) may be normal, especially in obese children, or may indicate cretinism, rickets, congenital syphilis, or Down syndrome. Absence of teeth is seen with congenital ectodermal dysplasia. Loss of teeth is seen in children with metabolic diseases such as acrodynia, xanthomatosis, histiocytosis, cherubism, gingivitis, and low-phosphatase rickets. Flattened edges of the teeth are usually seen in children who grind their teeth. The usual causes of tooth grinding are psychologic difficulties, mental deficiency, tiredness, and local irritation.

Malocclusion may occur without obvious cause or after premature loss or prolonged retention of deciduous teeth. It may be a family characteristic, and it also occurs in children with mouth breathing, cleft palate, mi-

TABLE 4-1
Chronology of tooth eruption

Primary		Secondary	
MAXILLARY			
Central incisor	7½ mo	Central incisor	7–8 yr
Lateral incisor	9 mo	Lateral incisor	8–9 yr
Cuspid	18 mo	Cuspid	11–12 yr
First molar	14 mo	First bicuspid	10–11 yr
Second molar	24 mo	Second bicuspid	10–12 yr
		First molar	6–7 yr
		Second molar	12–13 yr
		Third molar	17–21 yr
MANDIBULAR			
Central incisor	6 mo	Central incisor	6–7 yr
Lateral incisor	7 mo	Lateral incisor	7–8 yr
Cuspid	16 mo	Cuspid	9–10 yr
First molar	12 mo	First bicuspid	10–12 yr
Second molar	20 mo	Second bicuspid	11–12 yr
		First molar	6–7 yr
		Second molar	11–13 yr
		Third molar	17–21 yr

crognathia, or prognathism. One cause of malocclusion of permanent teeth is persistent thumbsucking after 6 years of age.

Dental *caries,* due to bacterial decay and disintegration of tooth substance, is difficult to detect without special instruments until cavitation occurs. Disintegration of the enamel may be detected with a sharp instrument, especially if tooth pain is present. The number of caries is decreased in children with Down syndrome.

Poor tooth formation may be seen with systemic diseases such as hypocalcemia, congenital lues, hypoparathyroidism, severe infections, and nutritional disturbances, including rickets and nephrosis. Defective enamel formation in primary teeth occurs in children with prenatal infections or cerebral palsy. Defective posterior incisors occur in older children or adolescents with bulimia.

Green or black teeth may be found after iron ingestion or after death of the tooth. Green teeth are also seen in children who had severe jaundice at birth. Red teeth are sometimes seen in those with porphyria. Brown teeth may be due to congenital defect in tooth formation. Mottled, pitted teeth may be seen following excess fluoride ingestion and some years after receiving tetracycline. Centrally notched, peg-shaped permanent teeth (Hutchinson's teeth) may occur in children with congenital syphilis. Mulberrylike 6-year molars occur in normal children but may also indicate congenital syphilis.

Usually, little *salivary secretion* is seen in infants until 3 months of age. Absence of salivation may indicate dehydration, fever, Mikulicz's syndrome, botulism, atropine ingestion, or congenital ectodermal dysplasia. Drooling is normal in children until 2 years of age and persists in those with injury to the glossopharyngeal (IX) or vagal (X) nerves. Gag reflex may be decreased.

Excessive salivation or drooling is seen in children with teething or caries, infections of the mouth, caustic ingestion, mental delay, mercury or phosphate poisoning, gingivostomatitis, familial dysautonomia, acrodynia, and infections of the salivary glands. A child 2 to 5 years of age who is in respiratory distress, sitting up, and drooling should first be considered to have epiglottitis.

Thick mucoid secretions are frequently noted following tracheal irritation. In newborns, unswallowed saliva or excess mucoid secretions are noted with tracheoesophageal fistula, probably due to aspirated gastric secretions with secondary tracheal irritation. Collection of saliva in the mouth due to swallowing difficulty is noted in children with ninth or tenth cranial nerve injury, especially that due to diphtheria, encephalitis, or myasthenia.

Tell the child that examination of the throat is not really painful but may be uncomfortable and that the examination will take "only a second."

Further examination requires that the mouth be opened further and the jaws separated. If the child is 18 months of age or older, trying to get the child to open the mouth voluntarily is worthwhile. One device is to ask if the child would like to examine a relative (brother, sister, or cousin) after leaving. Most children say "Yes." Give the child a tongue blade and say, "I'll show you how to do it. First you have your brother open his mouth wide. Then you look at his teeth, then you look high, and then you look low." Even though a gag is elicited, most children are not very angry.

If this suggestion fails, attempt to place the tongue blade on the anterior part of the tongue for a view of the tongue and palate. With the blade in this position, the child is not uncomfortable and usually does not resist patient examination. If the child resists by closing the mouth and gritting the teeth, carefully and firmly restrain the child.

Restraint can be maintained by asking the mother to hold the patient's hands and forehead. Place the tongue blade through the lips to the posterior teeth. Use small tongue blades for small children. Patiently, push the blade between the teeth toward the pharynx. Insert the blade with a slightly downward motion so that the tongue is pushed forward and the base of the tongue downward. Suddenly, the child will gag, the mouth will open, and in this instant, observe all the structures inside the mouth. At no time should the nose be pinched closed (see Figure 4-10).

To grasp well what you see, develop the ability to anticipate the normal throat structures and to retain an afterimage of the abnormalities seen. With practice, you will learn to prolong the gag, so that the structures can be more carefully visualized. Ask older children to breathe in and out through the mouth and carefully note all the oral structures that can be seen. If a large portion of the posterior nasopharynx cannot be observed, introduce a tongue depressor, and tell the patient to say "ah" or to breathe rapidly through the mouth. With this method, gagging can usually be avoided. Frequently, if the patient sticks the tongue out and breathes deeply, the tongue blade is unnecessary.

Note inflammation, color, swelling, and distortions of the *gums*. Redness, swelling, and tenderness of the gums are seen in children with gingivitis. Inflammation of the gingiva may indicate the presence of a systemic disease or vitamin C deficiency, or it may occur in mouth breathers or in children with erupting teeth, poor mouth hygiene, or poor dental care. Swelling or small cysts on the hard palate or gums in infants may be a sign of pneumococcal sepsis.

In a child with teeth, a black line along the margin of the gum may signify heavy metal poisoning. However, a melanotic line of the gums themselves is found in normal black infants. The gums near the teeth are purple and bleed easily in children with scurvy. The gums may also bleed easily in children with other bleeding diseases such as leukemia or chronic leukopenia, with poor oral hygiene, and sometimes in apparently normal children. The gums in children with herpetic stomatitis appear to be painted with a bright red pencil and are swollen and tender. Generalized hypertrophy of the gums is seen in mouth breathers, in children receiving phenytoin with phenytoin sensitivity, in children with hereditary gingival fibromatosis, and with many vitamin deficiency states. Pinpoint inflamed elevations from which pus can be expressed with the tongue depressor are characteristic of root abscess of the tooth.

In the young infant, epithelial pearls or retention cysts are found in or near the midline of the gums. These cysts have no clinical significance and usually disappear spontaneously when the infant is 2 to 3 months of age. White patches on the cheeks or lips in the older child that are asymptomatic may represent ectopic sebaceous glands (Fordyce's spots).

Next, inspect the *buccal mucosa*. In the young infant, look especially for thrush, small white patches that do not scrape off when rubbed. Patches that scrape off are usually due to milk or other ingested white food. Bluish-white scattered spots about the size of a grain of sand on the buccal mucosa at the level of the lower teeth and within the lower lip are characteristic of Koplik's spots. These spots usually indicate measles. Red spots 1 to 3 mm in diameter over the buccal mucosa and palate are characteristic of Forschheimer's sign, frequently an early indication of German measles. Vesicles on the buccal mucosa, especially if surrounded by a red line, are usually due to herpes simplex. If found on the posterior pharynx, similar vesicles usually indicate herpangina due to coxsackievirus infection. Pale red spots may cover the buccal mucosa in measles and other viral diseases and are the enanthems of the diseases with skin exanthems. Whitish ulcers occur with folic acid, vitamin B$_{12}$, niacin, or tryptophan deficiency. Painful ulcers may be a sign of erythema multiforme, leukemia, malignant neutropenia, and diphtheria.

Veins on the buccal mucosa are ordinarily not seen. Visible or dilated veins on the buccal mucosa or tongue may be an early sign of cyanosis or may indicate cardiac failure or local vascular obstruction.

View the *tongue*. Normally, the dorsal surface of the tongue is coated with conical filiform papillae; the reddish color is due to the blood supply to the papillae. Coating may signify mouth breathing or lack of motion of the tongue caused by debility in severe disease. Dry tongue is a sign of general dehydration. Unilateral atrophy of the tongue may be due to injury of the hypoglossal nerve.

Note *tremor* of the tongue as it protrudes. Fine tremor is seen with chorea, hyperthyroidism, and amyotonia congenita. Gross tremor may be seen in children with cerebral palsy. Fibrillations (slow undulating movements) indicate completely denervated muscle and may be an early sign of spinal muscular atrophy (Werdnig-Hoffmann disease).

Large red *papillae* resembling a strawberry or raspberry are seen with scarlet fever. White spots of thrush may be noted in newborns when they are due to maternal infection, in debilitated children, in children with hypoparathyroidism, and after prolonged antibiotic medication. A triangular red area along the outer margin of the tongue occurs in patients with typhoid fever. A sore, red tongue is seen with riboflavin or niacin deficiency states or with severe anemia. On the tip and sides are a profusion of red dots about 1 mm in diameter, the fungiform papillae. A uniformly smooth tongue with no apparent fungiform papillae is a sign of familial dysautonomia. Increased melanotic pigment of the buccal mucosa is seen in adrenal insufficiency, acanthosis nigricans, severe cachexia, neurofibromatosis, and pellagra. Occasionally, melanotic patches are seen on the tongue of children with polyposis (Peutz' syndrome). Black tongue may be congenital but has been described as a low-grade infection following penicillin administration or chickenpox. It also occurs in mouth bleeders, such as in patients with hemophilia. A bright red tongue without enlargement of papillae may accompany Kawasaki disease.

Geographic tongue consists of gray, irregular areas of the tongue and is usually due to unknown benign cause, but it may be related to febrile states or to allergy. Deep furrows in the tongue are seen in mentally delayed children and are due to biting of the protruding tongue. However, furrowed tongue is most commonly a congenital characteristic. Scars on the tongue may be due to previous convulsions.

Macroglossia (large tongue) is usually congenital. It may be an early sign of hypothyroidism or mucopolysaccharidosis or be due to a lymphangioma, cyst, or hemangioma. In patients who let the tongue hang out, the tongue may appear large. Protrusion of the tongue may also be due to a tumor or thyroglossal duct cyst at the base of the tongue.

Tongue-tie is caused by a very short frenum. If the tongue tip of the infant does not interfere with feeding or if the older child can elevate the tip to produce the sounds of *t, d, n,* and *l,* the condition does not exist. Cysts or ranulae are occasionally seen in the floor of the mouth near the frenum.

Paralysis of the tongue may be noted. The tongue protrudes toward the involved side in patients with hypoglossal nerve lesions.

With the tongue depressor still on the anterior half of the tongue, inspect the hard palate. Note color of the palate. Jaundice is easily recognised. Petechiae on the palate are usually due to any condition causing pharyngitis but may be due to other diseases that cause petechiae on the skin or elsewhere.

Congenital *cleft palate* is easily observed. Note if the cleft involves only the hard palate, the soft palate, or the uvula and distinguish it from the rare condition of palatal perforation. Perforation of the palate is seen in children with congenital syphilis after they are 2 years of age. High, arched palates are usually seen in mouth breathers but also in children with arachnodactyly and many other congenital disorders. Hypertrophy of the bone in the midline of the palate (torus palatinus) is usually an anomaly of little significance.

Advance the tongue depressor over the root of the tongue and press down. This usually causes gagging and is an unpleasant part of the routine examination. Because the child almost immediately resists further manipulation, this part of the examination should be done expeditiously, and you should know exactly what you wish to learn before causing the child to gag.

The first area that presents with the gag is the *epiglottis,* located at the base of the tongue. Note swelling and color. A swollen red epiglottis is seen in some children with laryngotracheobronchitis, especially when it is due to *H. influenzae,* and may obstruct respiration. A swollen pale epiglottis is seen with viral infections and allergy. Either a swollen red or a swollen pale epiglottis may represent a respiratory emergency. A congenitally large epiglottis or ulcers of the epiglottis may be noted. Lack of gag may be due to ninth or tenth nerve injury.

Next inspect the *uvula.* A very long uvula is congenital and may cause gagging or coughing. Occasionally, the uvula is congenitally bifid and may be associated with a submucous cleft of the palate. It may be absent, having been accidentally removed during tonsillectomy. Note motion of the uvula and soft palate as the patient is gagged or told to say "ah." Paralysis of the soft palate or uvula or absence of the gag reflex is an early sign of poliomyelitis and diphtheria, but it is also seen in disorders involving the glossopharyngeal or vagus nerves or conditions with masses behind the palate. Limited motion of the soft palate may be caused by hypertrophied, infected adenoids. A translucent membrane in the midline of the soft palate indicates lack of continuity of muscles and may be a sign of palatopharyngeal incompetence.

Look at the posterior *pharynx* for lymphoid hyperplasia, color, post-nasal drip, membrane, edema, exudate, abscess, and vesicles. Lymphoid hyperplasia is seen with any infection of the area. A red, inflamed pharynx is characteristic of any type of acute pharyngitis, but there are no good local signs to distinguish bacterial from nonbacterial pharyngitis. A pale, puffy mucosa indicates edema. Vesicles on the posterior pharynx, anterior pillars, or uvula surrounded by 3 to 6 mm erythema are a sign of herpangina due to coxsackie virus A infection. These ulcerate, and small ulcers may remain for 2 to 3 weeks. Small maculopapules on the posterior pharynx are also seen in other respiratory viral diseases.

Profuse postnasal drip indicates infection in the nose, nasopharynx, or sinuses and may cause a foul odor. A white membrane over the tonsils or posterior pharynx is seen in children with diphtheria; other bacterial infections, particularly Vincent's angina and β-hemolytic streptococcal infection; infectious mononucleosis; agranulocytosis; and leukemia. In diphtheria, the mouth smells "mousy," and the membrane pulls away with bleeding. The membrane in diphtheria is usually more confluent and spreads to cover more of the uvula and posterior pharynx than in the other infections. Indeed, a confluent membrane involving the uvula or posterior pharynx should be considered diphtheritic until proved otherwise.

The pharynx or throat is separated from the mouth by the anterior and posterior pillars. The palatine (faucial) *tonsils* are located between these pillars. Note size of the tonsils. Like all lymphoid tissue, tonsils are much larger during early childhood than later; therefore, statements regarding enlargement of tonsils in childhood must be reserved until you have examined many normal tonsils or until obstruction of the airway is obvious.

Crypts in the tonsillar tissue may indicate past infection; pus in the tonsils and peritonsillar abscesses indicate acute infections. The tonsils appear to be pushed backward or forward and the uvula may be displaced with peritonsillar abscesses. Peritonsillar abscesses occur more often in older children and are usually due to streptococcus infections.

In the infant under 2 years of age, erythema of the tonsils usually occurs with bacterial infections, especially streptococci, pneumococci, and *H. influenzae*. Purulent exudate or membrane suggests the presence of viral infections. In children over 2 years of age, some attempt can be made to distinguish bacterial from viral tonsillitis, although obtaining cultures of the nasopharynx is usually necessary. Yellow or grayish-white follicles are usually due to bacteria. Vesicles; nodules; punched-out ulcers; scanty or streaky membranes; and patchy gray, white, or yellow membranes usually indicate viral infection. A coalescent white membrane occurs with *Candida* infections. A coalescent adherent membrane is common in diphtheria. A bluish-gray membrane with ulceration is more common in children with agranulocytosis or other severe underlying hematologic disorders.

Tuberculosis and tumors may also cause enlargement of the tonsils. Definite unilateral enlargement of the tonsillar area is common with diseases such as Vincent's infection, diphtheria, and lymphoma. Enlarged, lobulated, red-orange tonsils have been reported in association with accumulation of cholesterol esters (Tangier disease).

Collections of movable mucus and pus may be noted in the posterior pharynx. This is usually postnasal drip and may be caused by sinusitis or infected adenoids.

Outpouching of the posterior pharyngeal wall is characteristic of posterior pharyngeal abscess. Examination of the retropharynx with a finger is usually necessary only if a retropharyngeal abscess or submucous cleft is suspected. Retropharyngeal abscesses usually occur in children in the first 2 years of life; they are felt as unilateral soft masses in infants who are usually quite ill and have noisy respirations and, occasionally, retracted necks.

Single ulcers without generalized symptoms are canker sores. A recurrent type of canker sore may occur with allergy. Sudden swelling of any part of the buccal mucosa also occurs with allergy.

Other types of stomatitis occurring on the mucosa include vesicles of chickenpox, mucous patches of early congenital syphilis, and general inflammation with vesicles of the erythroderma desquamativum syndromes.

After examining the throat, break the tongue depressor in front of the child and throw it away so that the child knows that this part of the examination has ended.

Vomiting is really a symptom. However, when vomiting is seen, note the nature of the vomitus and save the vomitus if physical and chemical examinations are desired. Vomiting in the newborn may have special significance.

Overfeeding, food intolerance, and improper handling of the infant are the usual causes of vomiting during infancy. However, vomiting of recently ingested food in children may be an early sign of infection in the intestinal tract or elsewhere. Other common causes of nondescript vomiting include severe coughing, brain tumor and increased intracranial pressure, psychogenic factors, food allergy, chalasia, gastroesophageal reflux, poisoning (including lead poisoning), metabolic diseases (such as medium chain fatty acid intolerance), and abdominal epilepsy. A common form of severe vomiting is seen in children 2 to 12 years of age; it occurs periodically, is probably due to a combination of psychogenic factors and lability of ketone-producing mechanisms, and is termed *cyclic vomiting*. Vomiting with nausea before breakfast may indicate hypoglycemia. Vomiting without nausea or vomiting liquids but not solids, especially in the early morning, may be a sign of brain tumor.

Forceful vomiting in the infant, especially of curdled milk free of bile staining, may be a sign of pylorospasm or pyloric stenosis but may also be the presenting sign of imperforate hymen. Vomitus containing bile may indicate duodenal or jejunal obstruction, whereas fecal vomiting is seen more commonly in children with lower intestinal obstruction, ileus, or peritonitis.

Bloody vomitus is most commonly due to swallowed blood from the nose and upper respiratory tract or from the mother's fissured nipple in a breast-fed infant. It is also seen in children with hemorrhagic diseases including Henoch's purpura, after the ingestion of foreign body or poisons, and after severe vomiting from any cause. Occasionally, bloody vomitus is seen in children with gastric, duodenal, or esophageal ulcers; anomalies of the portal vein; or cirrhosis of the liver with esophageal varices.

LARYNX

Note the *voice* or *cry* for hoarseness or stridor, which may indicate respiratory tract obstruction. Stridor is due to obstruction in the airway. In the first 3 years of life, it is considered an emergency until cause is found. Inspiratory stridor generally indicates an extrathoracic lesion, and expiratory stridor occurs with an intrathoracic obstruction. If the obstruction is so severe that the airway cannot dilate, the stridor will be both inspiratory and expiratory. Low-pitched stridor, especially if accompanied by salivation or snoring, indicates inflammation in the supraglottic area. The cry or voice is muffled, and dysphagia may be present. During inspiration with glottic obstruction, crowing is high pitched, the voice is hoarse or aphonic, and pain is present. During inspiration with subglottic inflammation or obstruction or with vocal cord paralysis, high-pitched stridor with a weak cry and little hoarseness occurs.

Stridor associated with wheezing occurs with intrathoracic or extrathoracic lesions such as tracheal inflammation (croup), where it is both inspiratory and expiratory. A low-pitched fluttering sound that is best heard over the larynx is characteristic of laryngomalacia. Snoring indicates upper airway obstruction, such as large tonsils or adenoids or a mass at the base of the tongue. Grunting with respiratory illness may be due to chest pain or may be a physiologic response to maintain increased airway pressure during expiration.

Expiratory stridor is heard with subglottic edema, vascular ring obstructing the trachea, tracheomalacia, bronchomalacia, asthma, cystic fibrosis, and bronchopulmonary dysplasia.

In newborns, hoarseness or stridor is characteristic of hypocalcemia; congenital laryngeal, epiglottic, or subglottic anomalies; laryngeal tumor; thyroglossal duct cyst; and injury to the laryngeal nerve. In infancy, hoarseness or stridor may also be due to a vascular ring surrounding the trachea, hypothyroidism, laryngeal infections, and laryngotracheobronchitis. In addition to these causes, hoarseness may result from shouting, laryngitis (including laryngitis due to diphtheria or measles), tracheitis, bulbar poliomyelitis, tetanus, Gaucher's disease, retropharyngeal abscess, foreign body, allergy, and croup in older children. Unless good presumptive cause of the hoarseness exists, laryngoscopy is necessary. Hoarseness due to infection is more commonly found in viral laryngitis or laryngitis due to *H. influenzae* than in infection due to streptococci. A low raucous cry is found in cretins, and a growl is found in children with de Lange syndrome. A sharp whining cry is found in infants with severe gastrointestinal disturbances such as intussusception and peritonitis. A catlike cry is heard in some children with a rare chromosome abnormality involving a deletion of material from chromosome 5 (cri-du-chat syndrome). Nasal speech may occur in children with chronic upper respiratory infection, enlarged adenoids, deafness, and neurogenic or anatomical velopharyngeal incompetence such as that seen with cleft palate.

Laryngoscopy is not performed in the routine examination. If indicated, it is best performed in the small child with an electric laryngoscope of small or medium size with good batteries and light. The child should be placed in a supine position and should have an empty stomach to obviate aspiration of vomitus during manipulation. The head is held with the neck partly flexed by the mother. The child's tongue is held, and the laryngoscope is slowly inserted along the tongue to the base. Visualize the posterior pharynx and epiglottis and note their status. A redundant large epiglottis may be seen when it obstructs the airway.

Pass the laryngoscope over the epiglottis and pull the handle up slightly toward the patient's head until you see the larynx. You may note laryngeal spasm, edema, paralysis, stenosis, redundancy, and tumors. You may also see thyroglossal duct cysts at the base of the tongue and the subglottic area if the larynx is normal.

In older children who can cooperate, indirect laryngoscopy is less traumatic. Seat the patient, warm the mirror, grasp the tongue, and pass the mirror back to rest on the anterior surface of the uvula, pushing it upward and backward. With good lighting, you can see the larynx. The cords are best seen if you tell the patient to say "eeee." This is the best diagnostic method for examination of the larynx when it can be used. It is particularly useful in problems of laryngeal motility and should precede direct laryngoscopy if possible.

Listen to the young child *speak*. The child should speak a word or two at 1 year of age, and put two to three word sentences together at 2 years of age. Speech should be almost completely intelligible by 4 years of age. Delayed or limited speech occurs in children who are hearing or visually impaired or mentally delayed or who have neurologic or physical abnormalities of the vocalizing apparatus. In older children, note specific speech defects such as lisping or stuttering. Deep voices occur in adolescent males and in children with adrenogenital syndrome and sexual precocity of other types. A nasal voice occurs in children with large adenoids, sinusitis, or palatal paralysis. Slurred indistinct speech with clicking produced by the tongue forcibly hitting the hard palate occurs in chorea. Aphonia with ability to whisper may indicate hysteria.

NECK

The examination of the neck takes 1 to 2 seconds but may help in the diagnosis of many diseases. The patient should be lying flat on the back or sitting.

First, note the *size* of the neck. The neck normally appears short during infancy and lengthens at about 3 to 4 years of age. A short neck is also seen in children with platybasia, Morquio's disease, cretinism, Hurler's syndrome, and Klippel-Feil syndrome. *Webbing* of the neck is sometimes noted in children with gonadal dysgenesis or as an isolated anomaly. Marked *edema* of the neck is noted in children with diphtheria, local infections, cellulitis, other infections of the mouth, mumps, obstruction of the superior vena cava, and any of the causes of generalized edema.

Next, palpate the anterior and posterior cervical triangles for *lymph nodes,* described in Chapter 3. Observe or palpate other *masses* in the neck. Enlarged parotids usually extend down into the neck. Cystic masses in the midline high in the neck that are freely movable and move upward when the patient swallows may be thyroglossal duct cysts. Pulling the tongue forward causes these cystic areas to move. Fistula may accompany the cyst. Midline cystlike masses that do not move freely may be lingual thyroid cysts, sebaceous cysts, lipomas, or dermoids. Diffuse swelling of the neck with nonpitting edema (bull neck) is seen in children with severe diphtheria.

Next palpate the *sternocleidomastoid muscle*. A mass in the lower third of the sternocleidomastoid muscle generally indicates congenital torticollis. Torticollis without abnormality in the muscle may be associated with gastroesophageal reflux and neuroblastoma. Oval, cystic, smooth, moderately movable masses near the upper third of the muscle are usually due to branchial cysts and may be associated with fistula or may be attached to the skin with a small dimple. These are almost always anterior to the sternocleidomastoid muscle. Cystic hygroma, which is usually posterior and above either clavicle, and hemangioma are easily compressible. Transilluminate for cystic hygroma or lymphangioma. Other masses presenting include dermoids, neurofibroma, ectopic thyroid, and lipoma. Hard masses suggest Hodgkin's disease; lymphosarcoma, rhabdomyosarcoma, or other sarcomas; and metastatic disease, neuroblastoma, and salivary or other malignancies. The callus of a fractured clavicle may be felt as a hard mass.

Next, palpate the *trachea,* feeling first the most anterior parts with one finger and then going down both sides simultaneously with your thumb and index finger. The trachea should be slightly to the right of the midline. Any further deviation in either direction indicates mediastinal shift due to atelectasis (especially due to foreign body), effusion, pneumothorax, or tumor in the chest or neck.

A palpatory *thud* (or audible slap) may be felt or heard over the trachea and may indicate the presence of a foreign body free in the trachea.

Next, feel just below the thyroid cartilage for the *thyroid* isthmus and for both lobes of the thyroid just lateral to the thyroid cartilage. The thyroid in the younger child can be felt with the child lying supine. Place your thumb on one side and your index and second fingers on the opposite side of the thyroid cartilage. In the older child, it may be easier to palpate the thyroid from behind with two fingers of each hand on both sides of the thyroid cartilage. The thyroid is observed or felt to move upward when the patient swallows. Note size, shape, position, mobility, and tenderness.

Thyroid enlargement may be due to hyperactive thyroid, malignancy, or goiter. A smooth, enlarged thyroid mass indicates thyroid hyperplasia. Nodules in the thyroid are usually adenomatous and may be malignant. Enlarged tender thyroid indicates early thyroiditis. A woody feel is characteristic of Hashimoto's thyroiditis. Bruit over the thyroid is common with thyroid enlargement.

Goiter with hypothyroidism may be due to antithyroid drugs or foods, Hashimoto's thyroiditis, enzymatic defect in hormone synthesis, or a deficit in iodine. Hypothyroidism without goiter may be hereditary, congenital, or familial or may be due to pituitary disease, sarcoid, or xanthomatosis.

Observe the *vessels* of the neck. Enlarged veins or abnormal venous pulsations may be due to increased venous pressure, which may be caused by heart failure, pericarditis, or masses in the mediastinum. Pulsation of the carotids may sometimes be seen in children, usually after exercise or emotional upset, but may indicate aortic insufficiency, anemia, hypertension, or patent ductus arteriosus. Venous pulsations in the neck in the upright child are always abnormal. In contrast to arterial pulsation, venous pulsations are obliterated by light jugular compression. Distended neck veins do not occur in patients with severe liver disease unless heart disease is also present. When heart failure is suspected, press on the liver. If the jugular veins become prominent (the hepatojugular reflux), failure is present. This sign may be misleading in the very young because they perform Valsalva's maneuver on abdominal pressure, making the jugular veins stand out. If the jugular veins do not fill on liver pressure, the venous system is not patent. This is a sign of hepatic vein thrombosis (Budd-Chiari syndrome). Unilateral distension suggests an intrathoracic abnormality. Bulging and collapse with expiration and inspiration indicate wide swings in intrathoracic pressure during respiration.

Note two small venous pulse waves: the *A* wave coincides with right atrial contraction, and the *V* wave coincides with right ventricular contraction. A prominent *A* wave occurs in patients with cor pulmonale, tricuspid stenosis or atresia, and pulmonary stenosis or hypertension. No *A* waves are seen in patients with auricular fibrillation. The *V* wave is prominent in patients with tricuspid insufficiency.

Venous pressure can be fairly accurately determined by measuring the distance from the upper border of the clavicle to the upper level of venous distention in the neck with the child in the sitting position.

The *carotid sinus* may be massaged in those children who have histories indicative of possible heart block. This is done only with the stethoscope on the chest. The carotid sinus is best reached by following the carotid artery up to the angle of the jaw and covering the whole area with your thumb. Massaging this area, one side at a time, normally slows the heart 10 to 20 beats per minute. A greater decrease in rate indicates abnormal carotid sensitivity, a rare cause of syncope.

Auscultate the neck with the bell stethoscope. Murmurs may be heard particularly over the carotid area but also elsewhere in the neck and are frequently transmitted from the heart with organic disease. Distinguish the benign venous hum near the carotids from an organic murmur by absence of a similar sound over the heart. To-and-fro bruits may be heard over an enlarged thyroid. Other sounds in the neck may indicate other vascular anomalies. Listen on each side high along the anterior border of the sternocleidomastoid muscle, the midneck, the lower neck, and the supraclavicular space. Bruits from aortic stenosis murmurs are heard bilaterally low in the middle part of the neck or at the angles of the jaw, which are the carotid areas. Those of vascular insufficiency are usually higher and unilateral. Transmitted sounds from the trachea may obliterate these sounds, except during the clear interval between inspiration and expiration.

Finally, note *motion*. First ask the patient to touch the chest with the chin and to turn the head from side to side. If the patient is unable to do this, raise the head from the pillow with one hand and turn the patient's head from side to side. Resistance to flexion of the neck (stiff neck) is characteristic of meningitis or meningeal irritation; in debilitated children with these diseases, the neck may remain supple.

Stiff neck may also be noted with the viral encephalitides, tetanus, lead poisoning, meningismus, and rheumatoid arthritis. It is noted with pharyngitis, cervical adenitis, retropharyngeal abscess, subluxation of the cervical vertebrae due to retropharyngeal or peritonsillar abscess, herniation of the cerebellar tonsils with increased intracranial pressure, and degenerative nervous system diseases as part of their generalized hypertonia. Hyperextension of the neck *(opisthotonos)* is due to any of the causes of stiff neck of a more severe degree. It occurs with respiratory tract obstruction and is also seen in children with cerebral palsy or kernicterus. Brudzinski's sign, obtained by flexing the neck and noting flexion at the hip, knee, or ankle, is a similar indication of central nervous system irritation.

Obtain the *tonic neck reflex* by placing the infant supine and turning the head to one side. The contralateral arm and leg flex and the ipsilateral arm and leg extend. The head is turned to the opposite side and the position of the limbs reverses. In practice, the opposite flexion and extension may occur and the test may still be positive. This reflex is present at birth and normally lasts 3 to 5 months. If present after this time, brain damage should be suspected.

Inability to move the neck from side to side may accompany any of the previously named states and is seen also with congenital torticollis, the Klippel–Feil syndrome, and occasionally cervical rib. Neurologic torticollis occurs in patients with lesions of the spinal accessory nerve, causing sternocleidomastoid and trapezius muscle paralysis, or it occurs without apparent cause. Eye lesions, especially when vision is unequal, or labyrinthitis, spasmus nutans, and brain tumors may be accompanied by torticollis. If the patient cannot maintain the head elevated (head drop), consider early poliomyelitis or other muscle weakness.

Voluntary *tilting* of the neck may be seen in children with habit spasm, brain tumors, poor vision, or strabismus. Head-tilting from side to side may occur in children in whom the corpus callosum is absent. Head rolling and nodding may be due to habit spasm, mental retardation, eye or ear abnormalities, or chorea.

5

THE CHEST

MANY DISEASE STATES can be diagnosed by simply looking at the chest. Sometimes doing more than observing the hyperactive or crying patient is difficult.

CHEST

The order of examination of the chest in a child depends on the attitude of the child; some find it easier to listen to the chest first, before the young child starts to cry, and then proceed with the other parts of the examination, whereas others observe and palpate first and use the stethoscope later.

Inspection

Note the general *shape* and *circumference* of the chest. Obtain the chest circumference at the nipple line. It is normally the same as or slightly less than the head circumference for the first 2 years of life; then it exceeds the head circumference. In very sturdy children the chest circumference is slightly greater than that of the head, even during the first 2 years. Marked disproportion between head and chest measurements requires comparison with standards for the child's age. Disproportions are usually caused by abnormal head growth rather than abnormal chest growth. When the measurements are compared with standards, however, the cause of abnormal growth can usually be determined. In children with respiratory disease, measure the chest in inspiration and expiration. The normal teenager can expand the chest at least 4 to 5 cm. Less expansion usually indicates intrathoracic pulmonary disease.

In the premature infant the rib cage is thin, and the chest may appear to collapse with every inspiration. In infancy the chest is almost round, the anteroposterior diameter equaling the transverse diameter. As the child grows older, the chest normally expands in the transverse diameter.

A round or emphysematous chest in a child after 6 years of age suggests a chronic pulmonary disease such as asthma. A funnel-shaped chest, characterized by sternal depression, may be a congenital anomaly or may indicate adenoid hypertrophy. A short, wide chest is noted especially in short children or in those with Morquio's disease. *Pigeon breast,* in which the sternum protrudes, is noted as an isolated anomaly or may be noted in children with rickets or osteopetrosis. The *xiphisternum* may protrude and appear broken, but this condition is normal in the young child and results only from a loose attachment between the xiphoid and the body of the sternum. As in adults, note is made of the rib numbers to orient the examiner. The second rib attaches at the angle of the sternum just below the clavicles.

With the patient lying supine, swellings at the costochondral junction may be seen. These swellings or blunt knobbings form the *rachitic rosary.* Almost always a depression will be noted in the child in the region of the eighth to tenth ribs, and the bottom of the rib cage will appear to flare. The depression at the site of the diaphragm muscle leaving the chest wall is known as *Harrison's groove.* Unless the flaring is marked, it does not indicate any disease. Although it occurs in rickets, this type of flaring is also found in many children with any pulmonary disorder, in children who were born prematurely, and in many normal young children who have no obvious pathologic disturbance. Edema of the chest wall occurs in children with superior vena cava obstruction, mediastinal compression syndrome, or mumps.

Note the *angle* made by the lower rib margin with the sternum. Ordinarily this angle is about 45 degrees. A larger angle may be found in children with lung disease and a smaller angle in those with malnutrition and deficiency states. Note *expansion* of the chest. Most of a child's normal respiratory activity is affected by abdominal motion until age 6 or 7, with very little intercostal motion. Later, thoracic motion becomes responsible for air exchange. If the interspaces show much motion with intercostal muscle retraction, lung disease or peritonitis is suggested. Note whether the motion of the interspaces is restricted to one side. Less motion occurs on the involved side, and increased motion occurs on the opposite side of the chest with pneumonia, hydrothorax or pneumothorax, obstructive foreign body, or atelectasis. Inspiration is normally about two thirds the length of expiration. Expiration is increased with obstruction in the larynx or trachea or in intrinsic pulmonary diseases, such as asthma, pneumonitis, or cystic fibrosis.

These disease states and paralysis of the chest musculature also produce increased motion of the diaphragm. With normal respiration the chest expands, the sternal angle increases, and the diaphragm descends on inspiration; the reverse occurs with expiration. Paradoxical respiration is noted when the diaphragm appears to rise on inspiration and to descend on expiration. Paradoxical motion of the chest and diaphragm may be produced by any of the disease states mentioned, particularly pneumo-thorax. The side of the chest that is involved tends to collapse on inspira-tion and remains stationary or appears to expand on expiration. Paradoxical respiration is also noted in children with neuromuscular dis-eases such as phrenic nerve paralysis or chorea.

Observation can sometimes determine the difference between high obstruction and low obstruction. *Retraction* is chiefly suprasternal and se-vere in high obstruction, such as laryngeal lesions, but mainly infrasternal in low obstruction, such as infantile bronchiolitis. Retractions are usually less intense in lower obstruction. Diseases such as croup, congenital la-ryngeal stridor, stridor resulting from injury of the laryngeal nerves, diphtheria, and bronchiolitis; diseases of the abdomen such as peritonitis; and paralysis of the diaphragm also produce marked retraction above and below the sternum, with marked intercostal activity bilaterally.

CHEST PAIN

Cardiac

Mitral valve prolapse
Pericarditis
Coronary artery insufficiency
Kawasaki's disease
Aortic stenosis
Dysrrhythmias
Pulmonary hypertension
Dissecting aortic aneurysm
Takayasu's syndrome
Myocarditis
Embolism-thromboses
Vasculitis
Precordial catch syndrome

Noncardiac

Trauma
Muscle fatigue
Asthma

Noncardiac—cont'd

Skin infections
Collagen vascular diseases
Pneumonia-bronchitis
Pleuritis
Pneumothorax
Subcutaneous emphysema
Tietze's syndrome
Adolescent breast development
Cervical rib
Slipping rib
Scalenus-anticus syndrome
Tumor
Mediastinitis-pneumomediastinum
Sickle cell disease, trait
Leukemia, lymphoma
Gastrointestinal, renal conditions
Emotional affect
Poisoning

Note *asymmetry*. Precordial bulging may indicate an interatrial septal defect, other causes of right or biventricular enlargement, pneumothorax, or a chronic localized chest disease. Lung tumors such as Ewing's sarcoma, as well as congenital absence of the chest muscles, may cause asymmetry. Asymmetry is, however, most commonly found secondary to scoliosis.

Weakness or deficiency in the sternocleidomastoid or trapezoid muscles may result from injury of the spinal accessory nerve. Chest *pain* may be accompanied by tenderness and may be caused by extrathoracic or intrathoracic lesions or may be referred from other organs (see box), such as the abdomen, spine, or neck. Pain over the lower ribs may follow trauma: pull the inferior rib margins anteriorly. The symptoms will be reproduced because of "slipping ribs."

Note the position of the scapulae for anomalies such as Sprengel's deformity, winged scapula, and Klippel-Feil syndrome, which are described with the examination of the spine (Chapter 7).

BREASTS

Note breast development (Figure 5-1). Breast development normally begins before pubic hair development.

It may be difficult to determine whether a breast that appears large is hypertrophic or is truly developmentally enlarged. The hypertrophic breast usually has a flat nipple with a small areola, and the breast tissue feels soft. The developed breast usually has protrusion of the nipple, enlargement of the areola, and a firmness to the tissue underlying the areola. Redness, heat, and tenderness around the breast may indicate infection (mastitis). Ordinarily, do not palpate the neonatal breast, which is enlarged for about 1 or 2 months. Examine breasts during routine examinations after breast development begins, when breasts fail to develop, or when symptoms of problems occur.

In girls, normal breast development begins between ages 8 and 14. One breast usually begins to develop before the other and is frequently tender. With the patient in the supine position and the arm under the head, palpate in concentric circles inward from the axilla and clavicle to the areola for each side. Precocious breast development in girls is usually normal but of unknown cause (see box). Complete central isosexual precocity may be caused by central nervous system (CNS) defects or precocity from any cause. Pseudoprecocious breast enlargement occurs in corpulent children and is merely the result of adipose tissue. These "breasts" are softer than true breast tissue and cannot be distinguished from surrounding tissue.

Figure 5-1
Breast development stages during adolescence. Stage 1, preadolescent (elevation of papillae). Stage 2, "bud" stage (elevation of breast and papillae with some increase in areolar diameter). Stage 3, enlargement (no separation of contours). Stage 4, projection (areolae and papillae form secondary mounds). Stage 5, mature (projection of only papillae and recession of areolae). *(From Tanner JM: Growth at adolescence, Philadelphia, 1962, FA Davis.)*

PRECOCIOUS BREAST DEVELOPMENT

Central isosexual precocity

Septo-optic dysplasia
Hydrocephalus
Cysts, brain trauma, brain tumors (for example,
   hamartoma, neurofibroma, optic glioma,
   astrocytoma, irradiation, meningitis)

Pseudo-isosexual precocity

Granulosa cell tumor
Follicular cysts
McCune-Albright syndrome
Oral contraceptives
Adrenal feminizing tumors
Hypothyroidism
Hyperthyroidism
Marijuana, opiates, amphetamines
Stilbestrol ingestion
Prescription drugs (for example, digitalis,
   cimetidine, isoniazid, phenothiazines,
   antidepressants)

Measure and diagram all lumps and repeat the examination 1 week after menses. A unilateral lump immediately under the areola is normal in developing tissue. In girls 8 to 10 years old and in boys 13 to 18 years old, subareolar masses immediately behind the areola that are firm, smooth, discoid, and 2 to 3 cm in diameter result from hyperplasia. These *masses* usually regress within a year. Small, round, hard *nodules* in the breasts of children, as in adults, may be caused by cysts or tumors. These masses are usually both nontender and irregular; they may feel attached to the skin or grow out of proportion to the remainder of the breast tissue. Swelling, tenderness, heat, and redness in nodules are signs of inflammation (for example cellulitis or abscess) and may follow ductal obstruction, injury, or infection in a cyst; these signs occur more commonly during periods of increased hormonal secretion. Tender nodules with ecchymosis indicate trauma.

Painless, circumscribed, firm masses may result from fat necrosis after an injury. These mobile masses may be fixed to the skin and must be distinguished from those immobile, not so sharply delineated masses that result from carcinoma. Small, mobile, circumscribed, tender masses, which increase in tenderness during menses, may represent periductal fibrosis, cystic ductal hyperplasia, adenosis, or lobular hyperplasia. Bilateral lumpy thickening occurs with fibrocystic disease. Nodules that are nontender, firm, freely movable, and sharply demarcated are usually fibroadenomas. The long curve of breast tissue extending into the axilla enlarges with hormonal surges.

True gynecomastia in boys usually results from unknown benign factors at puberty but may be caused by tumors of the breast, severe liver disease, drug usage, and, very rarely, gonadal or adrenal lesions. Usually breast enlargement in a boy is caused only by adipose tissue, but it may occur with gonadal dysgenesis, Klinefelter's syndrome, or digitalis administration.

Breast development is absent in adolescent girls with pituitary failure, anorexia nervosa starting before puberty, gonadal dysgenesis, adrenal hyperplasia, or severe malnutrition. Record the stage of development (Figure 5-1).

Galactorrhea, a whitish discharge from the nipple, may be caused by pregnancy, a hypothalamic or pituitary tumor such as prolactinoma or craniopharyngioma, or by drug ingestion. A bloody discharge signals an intraductal papilloma, a purulent discharge suggests abscess, and a greenish-black discharge suggests duct ectasia.

LUNGS

Next, note the type and rate of breathing. A newborn, especially a premature baby, will normally have Cheyne-Stokes respirations, characterized by periods of deep and rapid respirations alternating with periods of slow, shallow respirations or no respiratory activity *(apnea)*; this should disappear by 4 weeks of life when breathing becomes regular. Various brain or metabolic lesions that depress the central respiratory center may cause Cheyne-Stokes respirations.

The *rate* of respiration varies from 30 to 80 breaths per minute (bpm) at birth, 20 to 40 bpm in infancy, 16 to 20 bpm at 6 years, and 14 to 20 bpm at puberty. Young children tend to have an abnormally high respiratory rate when even slightly excited, so estimation of true respiratory rate is best obtained when the infant or young child is asleep. A rapid respiratory rate, *tachypnea,* is found almost always in children with any type of respiratory disorder, and a normal rate usually indicates lack of acute pulmonary disease. Children under age 3 with upper airway obstruction rarely breathe at a rate faster than 50 bpm, whereas children with lower airway obstructive disease, such as bronchiolitis, frequently breathe at rates of 80 to 100 bpm. In young children, tachypnea may be an early sign of heart failure.

A rapid respiratory rate also occurs frequently in children with generalized or localized infection, fever, poisoning, salicylism, acidosis, or shock. A slow rate suggests central respiratory depression, especially that caused from increased intracranial pressure, sedatives or other drugs, alkalosis, or poisons. Slow, jerky respiratory movements or bursts of hyperpnea alternating with apnea (Biot's breathing) may be seen with CNS lesions involving the respiratory center, such as encephalitis.

Note the *depth* of respiration. Deep respirations are termed *hyperpnea*. Depth of respiration is an indication of the degree of anoxia present, the state of activity of the respiratory center, and the presence of acidosis or alkalosis.

In obstructive respiratory diseases, breathing is usually rapid and may be deep or shallow, depending on the degree and nature of the obstruction. In metabolic acidosis, breathing is deep; the respiratory rate is usually rapid but is depressed in alkalosis of long duration. Listening with the bell of the stethoscope over the mouth of a small child helps in estimating the rate and depth of respiration and frequently assists in diagnosing the degree of acidosis.

Establishing your own standards for depth of respiration is worthwhile. Examine a group of children ages 1, 3, 6, 9, and 12 months and 1, 2, 3, 4, 5, 6, 8, and 10 years in both the normal standing posture and in the supine position. During normal respiration, air from the child's nose will be felt a measurable distance from the nose. Record this distance for each age. Each figure, plus or minus 2 cm, can then be used as your norm. The author's measurements for these ages, when the patients are supine, are 4 and 6 cm for infants 1 and 3 months, respectively; 10 cm for 6, 9, and 12 months; 12 and 15 cm for 1 and 2 years, respectively; 20 cm for 3 and 4 years; 22 cm for 5 and 6 years; and 25 cm for 8 and 10 years. Increased depth of respiration is indicated by feeling the breath farther away, and decreased depth occurs when you feel the breath closer to the child's nose.

Recognize *dyspnea*, or distress during breathing, by observing flaring of the nares and intercostal spaces, cyanosis, suprasternal and infrasternal retraction, and rapid respiratory rate. Try to note whether the distress is mainly inspiratory or expiratory; inspiratory distress occurs more frequently with high obstructions, and expiratory distress occurs with low obstructions. Distress in tracheal obstruction is both inspiratory and expiratory. Dyspnea may also occur with exercise, pain, fright, anemia, cardiovascular disorders, and hyperthyroidism.

Dyspnea is usually increased by exercise and forms the basis of the *exercise tolerance test*. If limitation of exercising ability is suspected, some type of graded measurement of this ability is desirable. Usually, children of various ages can be asked to run about or up and down stairs and are then compared with their peers for the development of dyspnea. Dyspnea that occurs too soon indicates any state that may cause anoxia or causes such as lack of habit of exercise, obesity, or emotional distress. Exercise of the arms causes more dyspnea than an equivalent amount of exercise of the lower extremities.

Cough may result from intrathoracic or extrathoracic causes (see box), including pulmonary infection, postnasal drip, foreign body obstruction,

---

COUGH

Intrathoracic causes

Allergies, asthma, fumes, drugs
Cystic fibrosis
Cardiac failure, emboli
Foreign body in bronchi, atelectasis
Masses (for example, lymphoma, sarcoid, Wegener's granulomatosis, tumors)

Infection

Pneumonia, bronchitis, bronchiolitis
Tracheitis
Bacteria (for example, *Haemophilus influenzae, Streptococcus pneumoniae, Staphylococcus aureus, Mycobacterium tuberculosis, H. pertussis*)
Viruses (for example, influenzae, parainfluenzae, HIV, measles)
Protozoa, including *Pneumocystosis carinii*
Fungi (for example, *Histoplasma, Aspergillus*)
Mycoplasma pneumoniae
Parasites (for example, visceral larva migrans)

Intrathoracic causes—cont'd

Chlamydia (for example, *C. trachomatis, C. psittaci*)
Rickettsiae (for example, Q fever)
Hydrocarbon ingestion

Anomalies

Lobar emphysema, cyst, sequestration, vascular ring, tracheoesophageal fistula

Extrathoracic causes

Foreign body in ear, trachea, esophagus
Smoking
Tic, habit, emotion

Infection

Upper respiratory, postnasal drip, pharyngitis, croup, laryngitis, sinusitis

Anomalies

Cricopharyngeal incoordination, long uvula, laryngomalacia, immobile cilia pulmonary anomalies, cardiac failure, allergy, emotion, habit, or a hair or irritant in the ear canal. Expiratory paroxysmal cough followed by an inspiratory whoop in a child over 6 months of age or followed by vomiting in a child less than 6 months of age is characteristic of pertussis, parapertussis, and respiratory infection following pertussis. A loose productive cough is noted in children with bronchitis, upper respiratory infection with postnasal drip, and cystic fibrosis with pulmonary involvement. A sharp, brassy, nonproductive, barking cough, which sounds like the bark of a seal, is heard in children with laryngeal diphtheria, foreign body obstruction, croup, and occasionally, tuberculosis. The child with croup is usually 3 months to 5 years old, is in distress, and is in the supine position. A tight, nonproductive cough is heard with pneumonia. A staccato cough suggests chlamydial infection.

Cough is usually nonproductive in children, even with tuberculosis or bronchiectasis, and *expectoration* is rare. Hemoptysis may indicate foreign body obstruction, tuberculosis, other pulmonary infections, trauma, tumors, heart disease, or bleeding from high in the respiratory tract; purulent sputum may occur in children with chronic pulmonary disease. A dry, irritative, persistent cough is heard in children with measles, tracheitis, or laryngitis.

The *cough reflex* can usually be elicited by examining the throat or by placing your finger in the suprasternal notch and pressing, which causes the child to gag. The cough reflex may be depressed in children with mental retardation, debilitating disease, and paralysis of the respiratory musculature and in those who have received sedatives or cough depressants.

Palpation

Palpation in children is performed by placing the palm of the hand lightly but firmly on the chest and feeling with the palm and fingertips. Palpate the entire chest. Palpation confirms your observation of the chest wall, such as position of scapulae, position or fracture of clavicles, asymmetry of the chest, and the presence of rosary, Harrison's groove, breast tissue, and axillary lymph nodes. Note any masses or areas of *tenderness*. A *thud* is occasionally palpated high on the chest as the patient breathes. This is a sign of foreign body in the trachea. Palpation of the heart is discussed later.

Tactile fremitus is easily determined by palpating the chest wall in children who are crying, who can cooperate by speaking, or who can be asked their name. Fremitus, when obtainable, is usually felt over the entire chest as a tingling sensation. Decrease in vocal fremitus suggests the presence of airway obstruction or may indicate pleural effusion. When the patient does not make vocal sounds, fremitus is normally absent, but it is frequently felt in children who have been crying and signifies a partial movable obstruction to the passage of air. Tactile fremitus is especially valuable in distinguishing the presence of mucus high in the respiratory tract, where fremitus is very coarse, from lower respiratory tract infection, where it is absent. Fremitus is a poor sign for distinguishing pneumonia, atelectasis, or space-taking lesions in a child.

Palpate the rib interspaces for retraction or *paralysis* of the intercostal muscles. Intercostal retraction is caused from increased work of breathing. Intercostal bulging during expiration indicates expiratory obstruction.

Decreased motion of the interspaces may indicate paralysis of the intercostal muscles, decreased respiratory activity, or, if unilateral, any of the causes of decreased respiration of one side of the chest. Subcostal retraction' of the diaphragm with hyperinflation of the chest suggests air trapping. *Pulsation* of the rib vessels from coarctation of the aorta almost never occurs in childhood. Pericardial or pleural friction rubs can occasionally be palpated and feel like fine vibrations. A crackling sensation under your fingers may result from subcutaneous emphysema or a bone fracture.

The axillary lymph nodes are palpated best by bringing the palm of your hand flat into the axilla with the patient's arm hanging freely at the side. A slight rubbing motion will indicate the size of the glands. Normally, several glands up to 3 mm in diameter will be felt in all children. Abnormalities of these nodes are described in the section on lymph nodes (Chapter 3).

Percussion

In percussion of the chest, use direct and indirect methods. In the direct method (Figure 5-2) the chest wall is tapped lightly with either the index or the middle finger. Every half inch of the chest is percussed quickly. This method is rapid, gentle, and informative but requires considerable practice.

When the indirect method of percussion is used, place a finger of one hand firmly on the chest wall; use the index or middle finger of the other hand as the percussing hammer and cover the same areas. The bases for good indirect percussion are (1) the nonpercussing finger must be pressed *firmly* against the chest wall; (2) no other fingers should touch the chest wall; (3) the patient should be sitting, standing, or lying flat on the back or abdomen; and (4) the percussing finger should move like a piano ham-

Figure 5-2
Direct percussion.

mer, with a very loose hinge-joint action at the wrist. Because the chest wall is thinner and the muscles are smaller, the chest seems more resonant in children than in adults. Therefore accurate information is much easier to attain by examining the chest of a child than that of an adult. If you percuss too vigorously, however, vibrations over a large area may obscure localized areas of dullness.

Posteriorly, percuss from the shoulders down to dullness at the level of the eighth to tenth ribs, where the diaphragm causes a change in the note. It is important that the head be in the midline position facing directly forward during this part of the examination. If the neck is twisted, aeration is not equal, and spurious dullness may be detected. The top of the diaphragm will usually be located at about the level of the apex of the costovertebral angle. Anteriorly, tap from just below the clavicle to the level of dullness. Percuss the sides of the chest from the axillae downward. Then, starting at the lower margin of the lung fields posteriorly and the upper abdomen anteriorly, determine the lower margins and the mobility of the diaphragm. It is generally useful to begin percussing in the areas where you expect resonance and continue to where dullness is expected. This is especially important over the area of the heart.

You will find a decreased percussion note, or *dullness*, over the scapulae, diaphragm, liver, and heart. Demarcate these areas. Normally the top of the liver is percussed anteriorly at about the level of the sixth rib from the midaxillary line to the sternum. The lower edge of the lung or the top of the diaphragm is usually percussed to the level of the eighth to tenth ribs posteriorly on both sides. Anteriorly, the diaphragm usually cannot be percussed below the level of the liver on the right. Occasionally a distended stomach will cause hyperresonance on the left, so you may have difficulty delineating the level of the diaphragm. Fortunately, most children have an indentation of the ribs at the attachment of the diaphragm to help indicate where dullness is expected. Usually the diaphragm is also percussed anteriorly at the level of the eighth to the tenth rib. In all these areas the diaphragm will usually move, as determined by changing dullness, one to two rib spaces between inspiration and expiration. In the child under 2 years of age, this motion is very difficult to determine by percussion.

These normal areas of percussion dullness may be altered as follows: liver dullness may be at a higher level than the sixth rib in conditions causing liver enlargement, elevation of the liver as in abdominal distention, or with atelectasis of the lobes of the right lung. The liver will be percussed at the level of the sixth rib on the left in dextrocardia with levorotation of the liver or with situs inversus. The diaphragm will be higher than normal in conditions causing collapse of the lungs or distention of the abdomen and will be lower than normal in conditions causing emphysema of the lungs with masses or space-taking lesions in the chest.

The mediastinum in children is usually percussed as the area of cardiac dullness. On rare occasions a broadened area of dullness above or at the level of the base of the heart may be caused by the thymus. Though this is without significance, note any broadening of the mediastinum, since it may indicate presence of other masses. Heart size will be altered by conditions altering the heart, which are described later, as well as by conditions causing a shift in the dullness of the heart or mediastinum. Localized areas of decreased resonance, dullness, or flatness may be found in children with consolidation of the lung, such as pneumonia; with lung collapse, or atelectasis; with increased fluid in the lung, such as pulmonary edema; or with accumulation of fluid in the pleural space, such as pleural effusion or empyema. Left effusion more likely results from pancreatic disease. Right effusion is more likely caused by heart failure or ovarian disease. Dull areas in the chest may be attributed to the presence of tumors. Dullness below the angle of the left scapula may occur with pericardial effusion (Ewart's or Pins' sign).

Hyperresonance of the chest is caused by an increase in the amount of air in the chest. It is found most commonly in children with emphysema and is usually accompanied by a lowered diaphragm. Localized hyperresonance may also indicate the presence of free air in the chest (such as pneumothorax) or the presence of loculated air (such as lung cyst or abscess, obstructive foreign body, or diaphragmatic hernia). Increase in resonance over the area of the liver may indicate the presence of a ruptured abdominal viscus.

Auscultation

During auscultation, listen for breath sounds, rales, rhonchi, and extraneous sounds. Especially during auscultation the child should be totally flat or totally erect, since even a slight turning of the head may decrease the breath sounds and suggest severe pathologic states. Because of the small size of the patient's chest and the desire to localize pathologic findings and to avoid the scratch sounds made by chest hair, the small bell stethoscope is most satisfactory for auscultation in children. The inside of the stethoscope should be clean, the tubing intact, well fitting, and about 45 cm long. Warm the stethoscope before use and press it firmly against the chest wall, or sounds that are artifacts will be heard. A tight fit of the stethoscope with the chest is usually easier if the bell is placed in the interspaces rather than over the ribs. Auscultate the entire chest, including the axillary areas. Children's fingers must sometimes be restrained from touching the tubing during this part of the examination because touching the tubing also makes extraneous sounds. If the stethoscope is not firmly on the chest, nothing will be heard!

Because of the thinness of the chest wall, *breath sounds* may seem much louder in children than in adults. Inspiration is three times as long as expiration with vesicular sounds, twice as long with bronchovesicular; expiration is slightly longer with bronchial sounds, and inspiration and expiration are about equal with sounds originating from the trachea. Breath sounds in a child are almost all bronchovesicular or even bronchial, so sound quality offers little help in diagnosis. Decreased breath sounds indicate decreased air flow and are noted especially in children with bronchopneumonia, atelectasis, pleural effusion, pneumothorax, and empyema. Increased breath sounds are sometimes heard with resolving pneumonia. Bronchial breath sounds may be heard over areas of consolidation in the older child. Auscultate the area over the mediastinum in the midline both anteriorly and posteriorly. Normally you will hear no breath sounds over the sternum or vertebrae. Increased breath sounds will be heard in these areas in the presence of consolidation, foreign body, or tumor.

Inspiratory *rales* are usually heard as fine crackles. They may be scattered over the entire chest in infants and children with bronchiolitis, bronchopneumonia, or atelectasis. Rales heard exclusively in the upper part of the chest are more commonly associated with cystic fibrosis. Rales in the lower chest are more common in children with heart failure. Rales heard only late in inspiration are more indicative of interstitial lung disease such as fibrosing alveolitis.

Frequently you will hear inspiratory rales only at the very end of inspiration or only after deep inspiration. The crying child inspires deeply before each cry, so auscultation may be quite informative during crying. Instruct slightly older children to blow against your hand, or tell them to blow out the otoscope light or to blow on a pinwheel; they will usually inspire deeply before blowing. Instruct still older children to breathe deeply through the mouth, especially if you demonstrate this type of breathing.

Expiratory rales are usually heard as crackles during expiration. They are prominent in bronchiolitis, cystic fibrosis, asthma, and foreign body aspiration. Fine rales are heard with pulmonary edema. Rales are mainly expiratory with intrathoracic obstruction to air flow, inspiratory with extrathoracic obstruction, or both with severe obstruction either in or outside the chest.

The presence of fine rales may be clarified in children, as in adults, by having the patient cough at the end of expiration. Usually you should demonstrate exactly the procedure you expect the child to perform. Even small children can sometimes be induced to cough in this manner. Rales that disappear after coughing usually have no significance.

Pleural *friction rub* is a coarse grating sound heard through the stethoscope with each respiration, as if it were close to your ear. It occurs occasionally with pneumonia, lung abscess, tuberculosis, or empyema. A loud slap may be heard high on the chest in a child with a tracheal foreign body obstruction. A crunching sound near the heart and synchronous with the heartbeat occurs with left pneumothorax (Hamman's sign).

Rhonchi caused by crying or upper respiratory infection may be inspiratory or expiratory and are coarse sounds. They can best be distinguished from rales by tactile fremitus or by holding the bell stethoscope over the mouth and comparing the sounds from the mouth with those over the chest. If similar, the sounds are originating high in the respiratory tract near the larynx. Any sound, especially if musical, that sounds the same over different areas of the chest almost invariably arises from the larynx or high in the trachea.

Wheezes are produced by airflow through compromised larger airways and usually sound more musical or sonorous than rales or rhonchi. Wheezes are heard more commonly in expiration than in inspiration and usually indicate partial obstruction during the expiratory phase. Inspiratory wheezes usually are heard in children with high obstruction, such as laryngeal edema or a foreign body; expiratory wheezes are usually heard in children with low obstruction, such as asthma or bronchiolitis. High-pitched wheezes are associated with severe asthma. Absence of wheezes in an asthmatic patient is a sign of very severe disease. Tachypnea with rales but no wheezes suggests interstitial disease. Crunching sounds heard during different phases of respiration may be caused by subcutaneous emphysema.

Vocal resonance can be obtained in children if they are induced to count, speak, or tell their names repeatedly. Increased resonance may indicate consolidation, and decreased resonance may indicate obstruction to flow of air.

Peristalsis is frequently heard over the left lower chest anteriorly because of the proximity of the bowel. However, peristalsis in the chest, particularly on the left side, may be a cardinal sign of diaphragmatic hernia. Murmur or bruits over the posterior lungs may be vascular or may occur with a sequestered lobe of the lung.

HEART

Soft is the heart of a child.
Do not harden it.

Glenconner

Certain basic information must be part of every examination of the heart: rate, *rhythm, size,* shape, *quality* of sounds, *murmurs* and *thrills, femoral pulses,* and *blood pressure.* In the routine examination of the heart, it is advantageous to evaluate the patient in several different positions if possible.

Pulse

Palpate the radial, femoral, and carotid pulses in the young child and the tibial pulse in the older child. Absent femoral pulse indicates coarctation of the aorta; absence of the other pulses occurs with Takayusu's syndrome or later stages of diabetes.

The normal pulse rate varies from 70 to 170 bpm at birth to 120 to 140 bpm shortly after birth. Rates of 80 to 140 bpm at 1 year, 80 to 130 bpm at 2 years, 80 to 120 bpm at 3 years and 70 to 115 bpm after 3 years are within normal limits. By age 10 the normal rate decreases to 90 bpm and in adolescence 60 to 80 bpm. Boys generally have slower rates than girls. Increased pulse rate may indicate excitement during examination, toxicity, fever from any cause, poor exercise tolerance because of congenital or acquired heart disease, digitalis intoxication, hyperthyroidism, pheochromocytoma or neuroblastoma, and, rarely, other systemic diseases. After the age of 2, the pulse rate during sleep is usually 20 beats less than during waking. Almost always, the pulse during sleep as well as during waking hours is elevated in active rheumatic fever, any other active infection, or thyrotoxicosis. In rheumatic fever, in contrast to other infections, the increased rate is usually out of proportion to the increase in temperature. The pulse rate is usually increased by 10 to 15 bpm for each centigrade degree of fever. In children with upper airway obstruction, pulse rates of 140 to 160 bpm are common; in those with lower airway obstruction, rates may be 180 to 200 bpm or higher.

Supraventricular *tachycardia* with rates as high as 200 to 300 bpm is sometimes noted in children with congenital heart or acquired myocardial diseases or with toxic states. An idiopathic auricular tachycardia may be a cause of sudden death in infancy. *Pulsus alternans,* in which one beat is strong and the next weak, is a sign of severe heart strain. A slow rate *(bradycardia),* less than 100 bpm in infants and less than 60 bpm in older children, most frequently means some degree of heart block. In infancy it is usually associated with a septal defect, digitalis poisoning, severe sepsis, and, occasionally, hypothyroidism. In young teenagers, sinus bradycardia, especially with sinus arrhythmia, is common. Rare causes of slow pulse include carotid sinus hypersensitivity, hypercalcemia, hyperkalemia, increased intracranial pressure and, occasionally, acute myocarditis. The slow pulse rate sometimes seen in children with hypertension in acute nephritis may be related to an associated increased intracranial pressure. Slow rates may be seen in well-trained athletes.

Water-hammer, or Corrigan's, pulse is felt as an especially forceful beat resulting from a very wide pulse pressure. It is noted best over either the radial or femoral arteries. Capillary pulsations, or Quincke's pulse, noted most easily after you press lightly on the tip of the nail, also result from increased pulse pressure. A method sometimes used for eliciting capillary pulsations is the rubbing of the skin of the forehead vigorously for a minute until generalized erythema appears. Observation reveals intermittent reddening and blanching in children with increased capillary pressures. Both of these pulse types are found especially in older children with patent ductus arteriosus, aortic regurgitation, or peripheral arteriovenous fistula.

Thready pulse is a rapid, weak pulse that seems to appear and disappear. It is usually a sign of circulatory failure, shock, or heart failure. A dicrotic pulse feels as if it has a notch in it. You may find it in children with typhoid fever or other sepsis. The normal pulse has this notch, but it cannot usually be palpated. Pulsus paradoxus is a marked change in pulse amplitude with respiration. Take the blood pressure several times rapidly in different parts of the respiratory cycle. Alternatively, lower pressure in the cuff 1 mm/sec. Listen for the first faint sporadic sounds and the point where all sounds are repetitive and crisp. Normally blood pressure does not increase more than 10 mm Hg in expiration. Larger differences may be found in children with well-developed thoracic respiration. An increase of more than 10 mm may be a sign of cardiac tamponade caused by pericardial effusion or constrictive pericarditis. It is a grave sign in the child with asthma if the pulse pressure between two beats is greater than 20 mm Hg, and in the child with cystic fibrosis the increase reflects severity of disease process. Reverse pulsus paradoxus, a rise in blood pressure with inspiration, is caused by an increase in left ventricular stroke output as in hypertrophic subaortic stenosis or during positive pressure breathing.

Almost all children, especially young adolescents, normally have sinus arrhythmia. Occasional runs of premature beats or of extrasystoles are common in childhood and may have no clinical significance. Regular rhythm in childhood is not rare but, if present, may indicate active rheumatic fever or other active carditis. You will rarely see auricular fibrillation in childhood because its chief cause—rheumatic heart disease—develops in older children or adults after childhood rheumatic fever. Arrhythmias, particularly ventricular, may cause syncope and may be seen in patients with long QT intervals. Premature contractions that disappear after exercise are benign.

Inspection

In the routine examination of the heart, inspect the chest for precordial bulging, a sign of right-sided enlargement, and the visible cardiac *impulse* and its localization and diffuseness. Frequently the cardiac impulse is noted in the normal child or in a child who is hyperactive, thin, or excited. It is not visible in many normal children. If the impulse appears diffuse, it may be normal. The position of the impulse sometimes gives a rough idea of the heart size because it may correspond to the location of the apex of the heart.

Other observations made as part of the routine examination of the heart include the appearance of respiratory distress, cyanosis, edema, clubbing of the fingers, capillary pulsations, prominence of veins, and abnormal pulsations of neck and epigastric veins. The presence or absence of femoral pulses and the blood pressure also help in determining the status of the heart.

The size of the heart is the best indicator of the presence of heart disease. Measurement of heart size by physical examination alone may be difficult in childhood, but estimation can be made with careful inspection, palpation, and percussion.

Palpation

Palpation is useful in detecting the apex impulse (point of maximal impulse or PMI) of the heart. Although the PMI is an important physical sign usually indicating the location of the apex, a more reliable guide is the apex beat. This is the position farthest toward the axilla and toward the lower rib margin, which can be easily palpated. The apex beat is normally at the fifth interspace in the midclavicular line after age 7. Before this age the apex beat is normally felt in the fourth interspace just to the left of the midclavicular line. The apex is usually at a lower interspace and more lateral in children with cardiac enlargement; pericardial effusion and various lung, spine, and chest wall diseases may also displace the apex.

The apex impulse may be difficult to feel in children less than 2 or in children with pericardial effusion, heart failure, or emphysema. A forceful apex beat is felt in children after exercise or excitement or in those with thin chest walls, impending heart failure, fever, or hyperthyroidism.

Occasionally you can distinguish right ventricular hypertrophy from left ventricular hypertrophy by palpation. Place your palm over the sternum with your fingertips at the apex. Pulsation below and to the left of the apex indicates left ventricular enlargement; with right ventricular hypertrophy, you usually feel the impulse as a sharp tap or as a heave more medially. A sustained lift in the xiphoid region indicates right ventricular overwork. A slow heave suggests increased pressure work; a sharper hyperdynamic tap suggests increased volume work.

Usually the first (systolic) sound, occasionally the second (diastolic) sound, and in a failing heart a third sound (gallop rhythm) may be palpated. Occasionally the child will complain of tenderness when the heart area is palpated, which does not indicate that heart disease is present or absent.

Vibratory thrills and pericardial friction rubs may also be palpated. They are felt as fine or coarse vibrations, either continuously or during some part of the cardiac cycle. Record position of cardiac thrills and their timing in the cardiac cycle. Obtain timing by simultaneously feeling either the apex impulse or the carotid pulse. Thrills at the apex are more easily felt with the child on the left side; basal thrills are more easily felt with the child sitting up.

A high-frequency thrill along the left sternal border suggests ventricular septal defect; a low-frequency, midsystolic thrill in the second left interspace indicates pulmonic stenosis; a midsystolic thrill in the second right interspace suggests aortic stenosis; and a continuous thrill indicates patent ductus arteriosus. Feel also with one finger in the suprasternal notch. If it is very pulsatile, suspect patent ductus arteriosus or aortic insufficiency. A diastolic thrill at the apex is usually caused by mitral stenosis.

Percussion

Percussion of the heart, as with percussion of the lungs, may be performed by either the direct or the indirect method. Scratch-percussion is an excellent way of determining cardiac borders. With the stethoscope over the heart, make longitudinal parallel scratches with a finger beginning in the axillary line and move toward the heart at about 1 cm intervals. As soon as the scratches are over the heart, you will detect a change in intensity of the scratch sound through the stethoscope (Figure 5-3).

You may find a combined method of percussion and auscultation even more satisfactory for estimating heart size and shape. Place the stethoscope firmly on the chest just to the right of the sternum. Tap the chest wall lightly with your index finger, beginning in the axillary line and coming medially. As soon as the finger is tapping over the heart, an immediate intensification of sound will be heard.

The heart is usually percussed easily as a triangular area with one side of the triangle extending along the right sternal border from the second to the fifth rib, one side extending from the right sternal to the midclavicular line along the fifth rib, and the third side expending from the right

Figure 5-3
Scratch percussion. The stethoscope is near the sternum; parallel scratches are made down the left side of the chest.

sternal border at the second rib to the left midclavicular line at the fifth rib. Normally, the heart of the infant is usually more horizontal, and the apex of the left border dullness (LBD) is to the left of the nipple line.

The area of heart dullness may be altered in a child with a normal or abnormal heart size. You may percuss the heart at a lower interspace or more laterad with right or left ventricular hypertrophy. Percussion dullness to the right of the sternum in the third or fourth interspace usually indicates right-sided heart enlargement. In children with emphysema or space-taking lesions in the chest, the heart will be pushed away from the lesion; while in children with atelectasis, the heart will be pulled toward the side of the lesion. The heart is percussed on the right side of the chest in children with dextrocardia. The heart normally moves a little as the patient is turned from side to side. If motion does not occur when the patient is turned, pulmonary masses or adhesions may be present. This physical finding, however, is rare in childhood. The heart may be percussed far to the left in the second and third interspace when the child is recumbent, and it may be in the normal position when the child sits. This change of position may indicate the presence of pericardial effusion.

Small hearts, characteristic of patients with Addison's disease or constrictive pericarditis, are rarely seen in childhood. An enlarged heart is characteristic of almost all types of heart disease: congenital heart disease with heart strain, anemia, myocarditis, or rheumatic fever. Less common causes of enlarged heart include endocardial fibroelastosis, pericardial effusion, patent ductus arteriosus, hypertension in nephritis, tumors, glycogen storage disease, or peripheral arteriovenous shunt. Patent ductus arteriosus may be present with a normal-sized heart.

Try to determine whether the right or left side of the heart is enlarged. Right-sided enlargement, which produces precordial bulging, is characteristic of conditions such as interatrial septal defect, pulmonic stenosis, or in older children, mitral stenosis. Right-sided strain, in general, is more common with congenital heart lesions, though left-sided failure is seen with coarctation of the aorta, tricuspid atresia, endocardial fibroelastosis, glycogen storage disease, aberrant origin of the coronary arteries, or aberrant pulmonary veins.

Auscultation

Auscultate in a manner similar to auscultation of the lungs. Listen with the child in the sitting and supine positions. Use both the bell and the diaphragm over the entire precordium, with special reference to the valve areas as in adults: the areas listed (Figure 5-4) are the listening posts of the valve areas and not the true or anatomic valve areas. These areas regularly

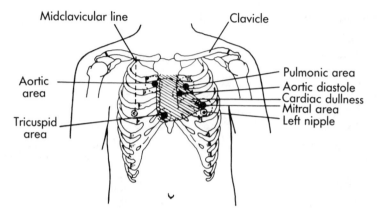

Figure 5-4
Listening areas of the heart.

include the mitral valve at the apex, the pulmonary valve at the second interspace to the left of the sternum, the aortic valve at the second interspace to the right of the sternum (and at the third left interspace for diastolic murmurs), and the tricuspid valve in the fourth interspace over the sternum. In addition to these areas, in children, auscultate just to the right of the apex and several centimeters to the left of the sternum in the third interspace (frequent sites of functional murmurs), along the sternal border (site of murmurs of septal defects), second and third interspaces several centimeters to the left of the sternum (sites of murmurs of patent ductus arteriosus and coarctation of the aorta), above the clavicles (sites of venous hums and transmitted murmurs), and in the axillae, along the left midaxillary line, and below the scapulae (sites of transmitted murmurs). In children, auscultation will usually give you a better measurement of the cardiac rate than palpation at the wrist.

Evaluate the quality of the sounds. The first sound, S_1, results from mitral and tricuspid (atrioventricular) valve closure and is best heard over these valve areas. When the first sound is *split,* the first component is caused by mitral closure. The second sound, S_2, results from aortic and pulmonic valve closure, the aortic valve closing slightly before the pulmonic. Splitting of the second sound is heard best in the pulmonic area and is common in normal children. The split widens on inspiration. Deep inspiration delays pulmonic valve closure and increases the splitting of the second sound (Figure 5-5). Learn to appreciate splitting by first listening at the apex when aortic valve closure is simultaneous with mitral valve opening. Then move the stethoscope up interspace by interspace to the

Respiration	A2	P2	Significance
Normal			
Expiration			Normal
Inspiration			
Wide split			
Expiration			Left to right atrial shunts
Inspiration			ASD, PS, RBBB, anomalous pulmonary veins, chest deformity
Paradoxical			
Expiration			PDA, AS, LBBB
Inspiration			Severe left sided disease
No split			PS, pulmonary atresia, truncus, tetralogy
(Split first sound)			Complete (RBBB), AS, PS, pulmonary hypertension, bicuspid A or P valves, coarctation

Figure 5-5
Second heart sounds (splitting).

pulmonic area where the pulmonic valve closure is most distinct; two sounds will be heard. A third heart sound, S_3, is caused by vibration of the left ventricle wall and occurs between the second and first heart sound early in diastole. Later in diastole, just before the first sound, a fourth sound, S_4, may be audible.

Paradoxical splitting, a wider split in expiration than inspiration, occurs with patent ductus, aortic stenosis, complete left bundle branch block or other severe left-sided lesions.

The first sound is best heard with the bell and the second with the diaphragm. In the newborn sounds may be normally distant or difficult to hear, although they should be sharp and clear. Distant sounds may indicate pericardial fluid, atelectasis, or another pulmonary disease. Sounds of poor quality, those which do not sound clear but are slurred or "mushy," are almost always characteristic of severe heart disease or myocarditis, usually with heart failure. In the newborn, both sounds are of approximate equal intensity. Later the apical first sound is louder than the second, and the pulmonic second sound is louder than the first in childhood.

A loud, snapping apical first sound is heard with mitral stenosis, left-to-right shunt, or conditions with high cardiac output; a decreased apical first sound is heard in early myocarditis.

Decreased or absent pulmonary second sound usually occurs with pulmonic stenosis, pulmonic atresia, or truncus. The pulmonic second sound is normally louder than the aortic second sound during childhood and is very loud with pulmonary hypertension. You may hear the pulmonic second sound better in the third than in the second left interspace in children. The aortic second sound is usually diminished in intensity with aortic stenosis and acute myocarditis. With aortic insufficiency the aortic second sound is often increased, but it may be decreased or absent. The aortic second sound is increased in children with hypertension from any cause. The tricuspid first sound may be obliterated with tricuspid regurgitation, a rare congenital anomaly.

Either the first or second sound may be split in any valvular area without causing concern, and a third heart sound is present in about one third of all children. Four criteria are useful in distinguishing split sounds from a third heart sound: intensity, quality, position heard, and distance between sounds. Split second sounds are of equal quality and intensity, are heard most frequently at the base of the heart, and occur with a very short interval between the sounds. The third sound is best heard at the apex, with a longer interval between the second and third sounds (usually with differing intensities and qualities), and occurs with mitral insufficiency or atrial septal defect. A fourth heart sound indicates decreased ventricular compliance as in fibrosis or hypertrophy.

Split second sounds at the base of the heart are common in children with conditions causing left to right shunts such as atrial septal defect, pulmonic stenosis, or right bundle branch block (see Figure 5-5). Splitting at the base is absent in children with pulmonic stenosis, tetralogy of Fallot, pulmonic atresia, or truncus. The wide splitting characteristically heard in children with atrial septal defects remains constant during inspiration and expiration.

Clicks are high-pitched sounds you may hear with valve openings. They may indicate aortic, pulmonic, or mitral valve stenosis or mitral valve prolapse. Low-pitched snaps in the mitral area occur with mitral stenosis.

Occasionally it is difficult to distinguish the third heart sound from a gallop rhythm, which indicates a failing heart. You may feel the three beats of the gallop on palpation; you can never feel the third heart sound as an impulse. Usually differentiation between the third sound and gallop rhythm is based on the presence of other evidence of heart disease, when gallop rhythm would be more likely than a third heart sound. Tic-tac rhythm, or embryocardia, exists if both sounds are almost alike in quality and intensity and are equidistant from each other. Although normal in the younger child, this rhythm in the older child may indicate a failing heart.

Pericardial friction rub is a grating to-and-fro sound heard through the stethoscope as if it were close to the examiner's ear. It is increased by pressure of the stethoscope on the chest or by the patient leaning forward. Intensity of the rub varies with the phase of the cardiac cycle. Rub usually indicates pericarditis, particularly that resulting from tuberculosis or acute rheumatic fever, and sometimes may be detected on palpation as a vibratory thrill. Pleuropericardial rubs are more common than pericardial rubs and are heard best in the manner described, but they vary with the phase of respiration rather than with cardiac activity. They may be confused with pericardial rubs, usually have no pathologic significance, and may be caused by the proximity of the heart and lungs but may indicate pleuropericardial adhesions. Sometimes the crunch of subcutaneous emphysema is confused with a pericardial or pleuropericardial rub.

Venous hum is a continuous, low-pitched sound originating in the internal jugular vein, heard sometimes over the clavicles. It usually radiates downward and has no pathologic significance but must be distinguished from a murmur. The hum is usually louder when the patient is sitting, disappears in recumbency, may be abolished by pressure on the internal jugular vein, and is louder on the right. Venous hums over the abdomen, especially near the umbilicus, are sometimes heard in children with cirrhosis of the liver or portal obstruction.

A difficult diagnostic feature in the physical examination of a child is the determination of the significance of murmurs. Many children have murmurs without heart disease, and occasionally newborns or others have severe heart disease with no murmurs. Systolic murmurs are those coming at or after the first and before the second sound; diastolic murmurs come at or after the second and before the first sound. Murmurs heard in systole are early systolic (regurgitant), midsystolic (throughout systole), or pansystolic (holosystolic). Holosystolic murmurs are caused by blood flow from a chamber with higher pressure to a chamber with lower pressure. Diastolic murmurs may be early (protodiastolic), middiastolic, or late in diastole (presystolic) (Figure 5-6).

The quality of murmurs is soft, harsh, blowing, or whistling. Grade the intensity of murmurs. According to one system of grading, a grade 1 murmur is the softest possible murmur heard. It is not heard in all positions, especially not when the patient sits up or after exercise. A grade 2

Type of murmur   **Examples**

Figure 5-6
Types of murmurs and examples.

murmur is the weakest murmur heard in all positions or after exercise. A grade 3 murmur is loud but is not accompanied by a thrill. A grade 4 murmur is loud but has a thrill. A grade 5 murmur is heard with the stethoscope barely on the chest. A grade 6 murmur can be heard with the stethoscope not touching the chest.

The intensity of murmurs alone does not indicate whether the murmur is significant of heart disease, though murmurs of grade 3 or louder usually do indicate heart disease. Following the intensity of a murmur over a period of hours, days, or weeks is helpful in determining the course of the heart disease. This is especially true in rheumatic fever and bacterial endocarditis, in which the quality of the murmurs may change rapidly.

Murmurs may "rumble" for a short distance around the site of their maximal intensity but "radiate" or are "transmitted" if they are heard with good intensity some distance away from that site. Innocent murmurs usually do not radiate, and they may change in character with phase of respiration or change in position—being louder in the supine position than in the sitting position. Innocent murmurs may appear or disappear during fever, exercise, excitement, or anemia. A diastolic murmur or a murmur that is transmitted or radiates indicates heart disease.

Cardiopulmonary murmurs are soft, high-pitched sounds caused by the apposition of the heart and lungs, occur always in the same phase of respiration, can be obliterated by changing position, and usually have no pathologic significance but may indicate the presence of pleural adhesions. Murmurs indicating pleural adhesions are usually short, high-pitched and squeaking, louder during inspiration, and project to the left sternal border. Murmurs originating from the left side of the heart are best heard in expiration.

Ordinarily short-blowing, early systolic or midsystolic murmurs of low pitch heard best in the pulmonary area (usually in early adolescence), pulmonary flow murmurs, or vibratory murmurs that sound like musical buzzing over the precordium (in younger children) are innocent. If these murmurs radiate, they usually radiate downward; if murmurs of mitral insufficiency radiate, they usually radiate laterally. Also, the murmur of mitral insufficiency is continuous during systole and is at or lateral to the apex; the innocent murmur, which is short, is usually medial to the apex in the general area where the murmurs of septal defects are heard.

A midsystolic, crescendo-decrescendo, loud, harsh murmur, "diamond-shaped," "ejection" over the pulmonic area is characteristic of pulmonic stenosis and is also heard with atrial septal defects or anomalous pulmonary venous return. This murmur is usually louder, harsher, and longer than the innocent murmur resulting from pulmonary flow. Peripheral pulmonary stenosis is accompanied by a soft systolic murmur over one or both lung fields but not over the heart. Pulmonic stenosis murmur may also be accompanied by a thrill and a systolic ejection click. A similar murmur in the second interspace just to the right of the sternum is characteristic of aortic or subaortic stenosis. This murmur radiates to the back. Atrial septal defect is distinguished by fixed splitting of the second sound, increased intensity of the second component of the second sound at the upper left sternal edge and at the apex, and an early diastolic rumble from tricuspid flow audible at the midleft sternal border. Murmurs of aortic outflow radiate to the neck and may cause a carotid thrill. An aortic systolic murmur, which varies in intensity, may indicate idiopathic hypertrophic subaortic stenosis (IHSS), a dominantly inherited trait. It increases on standing and may be associated with a mitral systolic murmur. A mid-blowing or late-blowing systolic murmur, frequently beginning with multiple systolic clicks, is characteristic of mitral valve prolapse. Murmurs of mitral valve prolapse may be "honking" or "whooping."

The murmurs of septal defects and pulmonic stenosis may be heard alone as isolated congenital anomalies or in combination, as in the tetralogy of Fallot. The pulmonary systolic murmur with a loud tricuspid valve closure, split second sound, and prominent precordial activity may result from anterior displacement of a normal heart as in the straight back syndrome.

Holosystolic murmurs are common with mitral or tricuspid valve incompetence and septal defects. In these the first sound is not heard. Detection of this murmur very early in systole distinguishes it from innocent murmur. Marked changes of murmurs with respiration are usually caused by right heart lesions (for example, tricuspid regurgitation) compared with left-sided lesions (for example, ventricular septal defect or mitral regurgitation).

Those diastolic murmurs that start loud and then diminish in intensity are decrescendo (for example, the murmur of aortic or pulmonic insufficiency). At the base of the heart, murmurs starting softly and increasing in intensity are crescendo murmurs, like the murmurs of mitral or tricuspid stenosis resulting from valvular disease or increased flow secondary to a left-to-right shunt. Presystolic murmurs are usually associated with active atrial contraction and stenosis of the mitral or tricuspid valve.

A continuous murmur in the second or third interspace to the left of the sternum that is widely transmitted is characteristic of patent ductus arteriosus. A hum or high-pitched murmur anywhere along the course of the aorta may be a result of coarctation of the aorta or, rarely, a thrombosis of the aorta. A continuous murmur in the right or left parasternal areas may indicate a coronary or other arteriovenous fistula.

Rheumatic carditis is a type of acquired heart disease. A harsh, systolic, high-pitched or soft blow, sometimes obliterating the first sound and lasting through systole up to the second sound or beginning in late systole with crescendo to the second sound at or just to the right of the apex, may be the first sign of carditis and is usually caused by mitral insufficiency. This murmur is usually transmitted to the axilla or back. Later, an early diastolic or middiastolic crescendo blow in the same area with a loud mitral first sound may indicate relative mitral stenosis—relative because of the disproportion of the size of the valve and the ventricle. These murmurs disappear when the carditis disappears. The murmur of true mitral stenosis is similar except that, in addition, early in diastole a snap is heard because of the mitral valve opening. A later snap in diastole occurs with pericarditis and must be distinguished from the third heart sound.

Late signs are the blowing diastolic decrescendo murmur of aortic insufficiency, heard best with the diaphragm stethoscope just to the left of the sternum in the third interspace. This murmur may radiate down the left sternal border. A systolic high-pitched murmur in the second interspace to the right of the sternum, transmitted to the neck with a decreased aortic second sound and often a thrill, is usually attributable to aortic stenosis. A systolic high-pitched murmur in the third left interspace, with a decreased pulmonic second sound, is usually caused by pulmonic stenosis.

Tricuspid murmurs are rare. Tricuspid murmurs are similar in character to mitral murmurs; a systolic murmur indicates tricuspid insufficiency, and a diastolic murmur indicates tricuspid stenosis.

The murmurs heard in the tricuspid area and the murmur of pulmonic stenosis are more often congenital than acquired during childhood. The murmur of aortic stenosis is frequently caused by a congenital lesion, and the murmur of aortic insufficiency is rarely heard during childhood, since aortic insufficiency develops late in the course of rheumatic carditis.

In general, the type of heart disease is not diagnosed by examination alone. First, make a tentative diagnosis by history and repeated observation and try to confirm or eliminate this diagnosis by examination and suitable laboratory studies. For example, children under 5 years of age rarely have rheumatic fever. Even if over 5 years, they should have other characteristic signs of rheumatic fever such as joint pains, subcutaneous nodules, chorea, or erythema nodosum. Even in an older child without fever or increased pulse rate, this diagnosis is not very likely, although it is possible. If a child has fever, increased pulse rate, and murmurs, also consider the diagnosis of fever with innocent murmurs or myocarditis secondary to infection elsewhere such as with nephritis, diphtheria, or tonsillitis.

In a child under 5 years, next consider whether the heart disease is cyanotic or acyanotic. Severe cyanosis at birth, which has been determined (as described in Chapter 9) in the newborn to result from heart disease, usually indicates one of the most severe congenital heart lesions such as transposition of the great vessels, truncus arteriosus, or tricuspid atresia. Cyanosis developing later in the first year occurs because of an increasing shunt from the right heart to the left, such as in tetralogy of Fallot in which the increasing pulmonic stenosis causes increasing right ventricular pressure. Cyanosis developing at age 4 or 5 may indicate

Eisenmenger's complex or pulmonic stenosis with septal defect. If cyanosis is not present unless the child exercises or cries, an atrial septal defect without pulmonic stenosis is suggested because the right-sided pressure is not increased until the intrapulmonary pressure is increased by crying.

The important noncyanotic heart diseases of infancy are toxic myocarditis from any cause, endocardial fibroelastosis, tumors of the heart, and, most commonly, patent ductus arteriosus and coarctation of the aorta. Patent ductus arteriosus has a characteristic murmur and high pulse pressure in the arms, very low pressure in the legs, and absent or weak femoral pulses. Other noncyanotic heart lesions, such as right aortic arch and dextroposition of the heart and aortic vascular ring, are diagnosed by examination and by history suggesting obstruction of the trachea or esophagus by an extrinsic mass.

The signs of heart failure in young children are not similar to those in adults. Early a rapid respiratory rate in the supine position is seen, followed by slight dyspnea. The liver becomes enlarged early and there may be venous engorgement and orthopnea; pulsus alternans and gallop rhythm, if present, are almost pathognomonic of heart failure. Signs of pulmonary or peripheral edema are found late in the progression of heart failure as the failure becomes more severe. Sweating may occur.

6

THE ABDOMEN

THE ABDOMEN IS frequently examined first in the younger child. The examination requires few instruments, but they may frighten the child. A thorough examination is impossible if the child is afraid or crying or if the abdominal wall is taut. Sometimes it is necessary to examine parts of the abdomen while the child is quiet and return to the abdomen later when the child quiets again. Warm the hands before examining the abdomen. If the child is ticklish, have the child place a hand over your palpating hand.

INSPECTION

First, inspect the abdomen, noting its *shape*. Ordinarily the abdominal musculature of the child is thinner than that of the adult, and the child has a lordotic stance, giving the appearance of a "potbelly." This appearance can generally be regarded as normal until the child reaches puberty.

Real *distention* of the abdomen is usually caused by air or fluid in the bowel or peritoneal cavity, but it may also be caused by atonic abdominal musculature, paralysis of the abdominal musculature, feces in the bowel, abnormal enlargement of organs, intestinal duplication, or tumors. Distention is frequently noted in children with pancreatic fibrosis, hypokalemia, rickets, hypothyroidism, bowel obstruction, constipation, ileus, or ascites. Transilluminate the abdomen with a strong light beam to differentiate cystic from solid masses in a child with an enlarged abdomen. Transillumination helps detect cystic tumors, bladder distention, and multicystic or hydronephrotic kidneys, as well as ascites.

Respiration is largely abdominal in children up to 6 or 7 years of age, and even after this age the abdominal wall usually moves with respiration in children lying supine and in pregnant adolescents. Peritonitis, appendicitis, other acute surgical emergencies of the abdomen, paralytic ileus, diaphragmatic paralysis, a large amount of ascitic fluid, or a large amount of abdominal air may be present if the abdominal wall fails to move with respiration. If respiration is entirely abdominal in the young child or largely abdominal in the older child, suspect emphysema, pneumonia, or other pulmonary disorders.

The abdomen is normally flat when the child is in the supine position. Occasionally, however, the abdomen will appear depressed or scaphoid. In the newborn this may signify a large diaphragmatic hernia with most of the abdominal contents in the chest. In older children, scaphoid abdomen occurs with marked dehydration or high intestinal obstruction. With pneumothorax, the chest is large and the abdomen, though normal, may appear to be scaphoid.

Observe the *umbilicus*. Normally it is closed and puckered, but hernia may be present as observed by protrusion of some abdominal contents. Umbilical hernias are common in all infants up to the age of 2 and in black children up to the age of 7. Hernias are especially common in children with hypothyroidism; Down syndrome; the chondrodystrophies; or large, chronically distended abdomens. Granulomas, ulcers, and drainage of the umbilicus occur in the newborn and are discussed later. If present, umbilical hernias and diastasis of the recti can frequently be observed when the child cries or coughs.

Diastasis of the rectus muscles may be noted as a protrusion in the midline, usually from the xiphoid to the umbilicus but occasionally down to the symphysis pubis. Ordinarily the protrusion is ½ to 2 inches wide; it is usually a normal variant but may be caused by a congenital weakness of the musculature or a chronically distended abdomen.

Paradoxical motion of the umbilicus is noted with unilateral or asymmetric paralysis of the abdominal wall musculature or of one part of the diaphragm.

Note the *veins*. In infants with good subcutaneous tissue, veins are rarely visible. Visible but not distended veins are usual until puberty in healthy children and are especially noticeable in malnourished children. Distended veins are seen with heart failure, peritonitis, and venous obstruction. Milk a vein toward the heart and away from the heart to determine direction of flow of blood in dilated veins. Blood flow from the veins below the umbilicus, normally downward, is usually reversed in children with obstruction of the inferior vena cava or portal hypertension. Diffuse epigastric pulsations may be normal or may indicate right ventricular hypertrophy with transmission of the pulsations through the diaphragm.

Next look for *peristalsis,* or *gastric waves.* Peristalsis is most easily seen if your eye is about at the level of the abdomen and a light is directed across the abdomen. Moving shadows will be noted in the presence of excessive peristalsis. Visible peristalsis is always a sign of obstruction until ruled otherwise. It may be seen normally in thin, small infants, especially premature ones. In infants up to 2 months of age, visible peristalsis may indicate pyloric stenosis or pylorospasm, but the type of obstruction cannot be distinguished by the nature of the visible peristalsis.

AUSCULTATION

Next, auscultate the abdomen and listen for peristalsis. It is better to auscultate the abdomen before proceeding with the examination, not only because you frequently forget to listen if this part of the examination is postponed, but also because manipulation done later may so alter peristaltic sounds that a true appraisal becomes impossible.

Peristaltic sounds are normally heard as metallic short tinkling. A sound may be heard normally every 10 to 30 seconds. Place the stethoscope firmly over the abdomen and listen carefully because the sounds may normally be of low intensity. Sounds may be increased in frequency and intensity simply by stroking the abdomen with a fingernail. They are high pitched and frequent in early peritonitis, diarrhea from any cause, intestinal obstruction, and gastroenteritis. Peristaltic sounds are absent in paralytic ileus and may be decreased to absent in children with early peritonitis. Listening to the abdomen and hearing the typical sounds of peritonitis may be the only way of detecting pneumococcal peritonitis in nephrosis or in other conditions where there is free fluid in the abdomen, since free fluid may give you the impression of a non-tense abdomen even though peritonitis is present. Rarely a venous hum may be heard during auscultation as a sign of portal obstruction. A murmur may be heard over the abdomen in children with coarctation of the aorta. Auscultate the area over the kidneys posteriorly with the bell stethoscope in children with hypertension. A murmur in this area may suggest constriction of one of the renal arteries.

PERCUSSION

After auscultating the abdomen, percuss by the indirect or scratch methods previously described. A tympanitic sound in a distended abdomen signifies that gas is present in the abdomen. Tympanites, or an unusually tympanitic sound, is common with low intestinal obstruction, air swallowing, and paralytic ileus.

A distended abdomen with little tympany suggests fluid or solid masses. When you suspect fluid, test for *fluid wave* and *shifting dullness.*

Fluid wave may be elicited in the following manner: The edge of an aide's hand is placed firmly along the midline of the abdomen. Place one of your hands on one side of the patient's abdomen. Sharply strike the opposite side of the patient's abdomen with your other hand. A wave is felt against your first hand, as if the wave arises from deep in the abdomen. Shifting dullness is most easily obtained by percussing and delineating the area of dullness with the patient in one position. Then, change the position of the patient and elicit dullness again. Slight shifting dullness is normal or may be found with tumors, but considerable shift usually indicates free abdominal fluid. Fluid in the abdomen (ascites) is found in children with chronic liver disease (for example, cirrhosis), chronic kidney disease (for example, nephrosis), tuberculous peritonitis, and rarely, heart failure or rupture or other leak of the abdominal lymphatics, (chylous ascites).

Solid masses will also be percussed. Frequently, a dull percussion note indicates a mass that cannot be felt. There is always dullness to percussion in the area of the liver, except if free air is present in the abdominal cavity.

PALPATION

Several methods are satisfactory for palpating the abdomen, though all methods should consider the comfort of the patient and yourself.

Distract the patient during abdominal palpation by using unrelated conversation or other means. Palpating the abdomen with the child asleep is especially helpful if an acute abdomen is suspected. If the patient will cooperate, the patient can be asked to take deep breaths and to flex the knees during this part of the examination. Palpation is best performed if it can be done in inspiration and expiration. Place one hand flat on the patient's back and the other on the anterior surface of the abdomen. First, palpate gently and *superficially,* using the upper hand for most of the palpatory sensation. Begin in the left lower quadrant and then proceed to the left upper, right upper, right lower quadrants, and middle. If a localized site of pain or tenderness is found, palpate this area after the other parts of the abdomen have been palpated.

Note first whether the abdomen is soft or hard. With a *tense* abdomen, there is a feeling of marked rigidity or resistance to pressure. A hard, tense abdomen immediately directs you to consider a surgical condition, any condition that may produce tenderness, or rarely, tetanus and hypoparathyroidism. In a crying child, distinguish between a soft and hard abdomen by feeling immediately on inspiration when the child may relax for an instant. If the child is tense and does not relax and a question of abdominal pathology exists, the child of any age can be placed in a warm tub. This act may relax the abdomen enough to feel masses or to localize tenderness or rigidity.

Note *tenderness* and the point of maximal tenderness. Frequently a patient will say an area is tender, and you may doubt the accuracy of the statement. In such a case it is best to touch a completely neutral area such as the thigh and ask the patient if that area is tender. Do not ask the patient, "Does this hurt?" unless the patient is old enough to be completely reliable. Rather, you can determine the site of tenderness by watching the patient's face, noting wincing, cry, and change of pitch of cry as the really tender area is touched. Note the pupils when palpating. When a truly tender area is touched, the pupils will dilate. Frequently the child with pseudopain will keep the eyes closed during the examination, but with organic pain, the child will eye your hand as you palpate.

When asked where the abdomen hurts, a young child almost always points to the umbilicus. Pointing to any other part may be more significant of pathology. Tenderness can be further localized by noting pain on *rebound*. Place one hand deep in the abdomen, away from the suspected area of tenderness and quickly remove your hand. The child may again complain of pain in the area originally under suspicion.

In general, even localized tenderness is not well correlated with underlying pathology. Tenderness in the lower quadrants may be due to such states as gastroenteritis, feces, obstruction, tumor, or rarely, Meckel's diverticulum with ulceration, torsion of the ovary, and torsion of the testis. Lower abdominal tenderness after a menstrual period may result from pelvic infection. Tenderness in the right lower quadrant with exquisite superficial skin tenderness may be caused by appendicitis or abscess; in the right upper quadrant, acutely enlarged liver, hepatitis, cholecystitis, pelvic inflammation, or intussusception; in the left upper quadrant, acute splenic enlargement, intussusception, or splenic rupture. Midline tenderness in the upper abdomen may result from gastroenteritis, coughing, vomiting, or gastric or duodenal ulcer. In the midline of the lower abdomen, marked superficial tenderness may be diagnostic of cystitis, but deep tenderness may result from the palpation of the normal aorta. Intraabdominal tenderness can be distinguished from muscle tenderness by asking the child to raise the head and then palpate. Intraabdominal tenderness is lessened, whereas superficial tenderness is increased by this maneuver.

Poorly localized areas of abdominal tenderness may be caused by pneumonia, upper respiratory infection, mesenteric adenitis, peritonitis, rheumatic fever, measles, crisis of sickle cell anemia, leukemia, allergy, acidosis, emotional crisis, other infections, or ruptured viscus. Disease in or near the spinal cord can cause referred pain to the abdomen.

If the abdominal wall is not tense, feel for the superficial masses. The enlarged *spleen* is usually felt as a superficial mass in the left upper quadrant. It may feel like a tongue hanging from the left costal margin with a sharp straight border and a notch on the anterior margin. Splenic enlargement is found in children with such diseases as septicemia; other infections; blood dyscrasias, including sickle cell or iron deficient anemia; thalassemia major; hemolytic jaundice; infectious mononucleosis and leukemia; lysosomal storage diseases; and connective tissue diseases. A very large spleen with less enlarged liver is seen with portal vein obstruction and neonatal hepatitis. It may be normally palpable 1 to 2 cm below the left costal margin in newborns (because of extramedullary hematopoiesis) and in normal infants and young children. Note its size and whether it is tender. Floating ribs are sometimes confused with the spleen on palpation. Usually you can differentiate by palpation or percussion.

The *liver* is generally palpable as a superficial mass 1 to 2 cm below the right costal margin, with a sharp border in newborns and infants. Note size, consistency, tenderness, and pulsation. The liver may remain palpable during childhood without pathologic significance.

Total span by percussion is about 5 cm at 6 months of age, 7 cm at 3 years of age, 8 to 10 cm at 10 years of age, and 9 to 12 cm at adolescence. If it is larger or more than 2 cm below the costal margin, the span may indicate such states as passive congestion, hepatitis, tumor or metastases, blood dyscrasias, septicemia or other infections, the reticuloendothelial or metabolic diseases, or pulmonary emphysema. Rapidly enlarging liver is an early sign of right heart failure. The liver edge is usually not as sharp in heart failure as it is in pulmonary emphysema without failure. Rapidly decreasing liver size may be diagnostic of acute liver necrosis. A thrill felt over an enlarged liver or a gurgling sound is found with hydatid echinococcal cysts in the liver. Friction rub over the liver occurs with pelvic inflammatory disease. Pulsation of the liver usually results from transmission of the impulse from the aorta, but quite rarely it may be because of tricuspid regurgitation or stenosis or constrictive pericarditis.

Other *masses* such as neuroblastoma, Wilms' tumor, duplication of the intestinal tract and urinary bladder, circumscribed collections of blood, collection of fluid in the uterus resulting from an imperforate hymen, hydrometrocolpos, and an enlarged uterus attributed to pregnancy may be palpated superficially. The spleen can be pushed medially, laterally, and upward if necessary to distinguish it from an enlarged left lobe of the liver. It may be felt superficial to the colon, distinguishing it from a retroperitoneal mass. Wilms' tumor may be distinguished from a neuroblastoma, since Wilms' tumor ordinarily does not cross the midline; however, it may be bilateral, especially in younger children. Ovarian tumors palpated in preadolescent girls may be malignant; after menarche they are more likely to be functional.

After superficial palpation, proceed in the same manner around the quadrants of the abdomen but palpate more *deeply,* using the posterior hand to push masses forward. The anterior hand pushes down so that the skin of the anterior abdomen is actually indented 2 to 5 cm. In children with ascites, it may be difficult to feel any masses directly. However, percussion may indicate a few areas of increased dullness, and palpation by *ballottement* should delineate a few of the larger masses. In ballotting (Figure 6-1), place one hand lightly above the area to be ballotted and one hand firmly below the area to be ballotted. With the ballotting hand, quickly flick the area. If a ballottable mass is present, a rebound sensation will be felt in the flicking hand, as if a ball had been thrown forward and came back.

In addition to delineating the masses already noted, look for certain special masses. For example, the tumor of pyloric stenosis is best felt on deep palpation after the infant vomits. This mass is usually located at the end of the stomach anywhere along the edge of the liver from the costal margin in the midline to the underside of the right lobe of the liver. The

Figure 6-1
Ballotting for right kidney.

sausage-shaped tender mass of intussusception can usually be palpated in the right upper quadrant. Other masses such as those caused by urinary tract anomalies (for example, malposition, hydroureter, and hydronephrosis) and the filled bladder may be palpated. *Bladder* enlargement may be attributable to anatomic urinary tract obstruction, voluntary control, embarrassment of the patient, or low spinal cord lesions.

By placing the index finger in the costovertebral angle and pushing up gently but sharply (as in ballottement), you can usually palpate about 1 or 2 cm of the right *kidney* and frequently the tip of the left kidney. The reverse procedure even more frequently allows you to feel the normal as well as the enlarged kidney: Gently elevate the abdomen of the child in the supine position with one hand, and place all the fingers of the other hand flat over the back of the elevated side so that the index finger lies in the costovertebral angle. Release the hand that is holding the abdomen forward; as the side of the abdomen falls toward the mattress, the kidney will hit the back of your hand. Enlarged kidneys usually indicate infection, congenital anomaly, tumor of the kidney, or renal vein thrombosis.

Remember that a few children have malrotation of the organs, as in situs inversus and congenital malrotation. In children who have had operations for repair of omphalocele and sometimes for diaphragmatic hernia, the organs are so displaced that it may be impossible to recognize even normal organs.

Every mass in the abdomen must be explained adequately before a patient can be considered free of disease. Occasionally, however, you may mistake feces in a child who is not even constipated or confuse the abdominal aorta with an abnormal mass. Palpate also for a diastasis between the rectus muscles.

Palpate the umbilical hernia previously noted. Note the presence of bowel in the hernia by palpating a gas–filled loop and obtaining the feeling of silk rubbing against silk on replacing the viscus. If the hernia cannot be easily reduced, make careful note of its size.

Obtain *abdominal reflexes* by scratching the skin of the abdomen with four scratches to make a diamond, the points of the diamond being the midline shortly below the xiphoid and above the symphysis and both sides of the abdomen at the level of the umbilicus. The umbilicus normally moves at each scratch. This skin reflex is absent in normal children under 1 year of age and in children with early poliomyelitis, multiple sclerosis, or other central or pyramidal disorders.

Next, palpate the inguinal and femoral regions for hernias, lymph nodes, and femoral pulses (Figure 6-2). *Femoral pulses* are best felt by placing the tips of two or three fingers along the inguinal ligament about

Figure 6-2
Palpating femoral area for femoral pulse.

midway between the iliac crest and symphysis pubis. With gentle pressure, definite pulsation should be felt by one of the fingers. Alternatively, direct pressure on the two or three fingers by the fingers of the free hand may make it easier to feel the pulse. Absent femoral pulse indicates coarctation of the aorta. Auscultation over the femoral artery may reveal a booming sound or "pistol shot," characteristic of aortic insufficiency or other causes of increased pulse pressure. A double sound (Traube's double tone) is indicative of the same conditions. A systolic and diastolic murmur may also be heard in these conditions (Duroziez's disease). Hernias are palpated in a special manner.

One of the favorite sites of determining *dehydration* in a child is over the abdomen. Pull up about 2 or 3 inches of the skin and subcutaneous tissue and quickly release it. If the creases formed by pulling the skin do not disappear immediately, dehydration is present.

Occasionally the wall of the abdomen feels putty-like in *consistency*. This may be normal, but it occurs in children who are chronically malnourished or dehydrated and in children with such diseases as peritonitis, tuberculous peritonitis, the lysosomal storage diseases, myxedema, and hyperelectrolytemia.

GENITALIA

Inspect the genitalia. Pubic hair stages (see Figure 3-3) are useful in quantifying development. *Urethral discharges* are always pathologic in childhood and may indicate infection anywhere in the urinary tract. A flaming red area around the end of the urethra may be caused by prolapse of the urethral mucosa. Eccentric masses near the urethra may be cyst, urethral polyp, papilloma, caruncle, condyloma, sarcoma botryoides, prolapsed ureterocele, or periurethral abscess.

With the child in the knee-chest position, inspect the vaginal orifice (Figures 6-3 and 6-4). In the preschool and early school girl the opening is about 1 to 4 × 3 to 8 mm, and in the preadolescent about 1 to 2 mm larger. Rough vaginal borders or a much larger orifice may indicate manipulation or abuse. Small tender ulcers may be indicative of herpes simplex or other infections, including other sexually transmitted diseases.

Adhesions of the labia majora in the newborn may be a congenital malformation or may occur in children with congenital adrenal hyperplasia. Imperforate hymen may be noted. This may cause hydrocolpos in the young girl or hematocolpos in the pubertal girl. Have the patient cough. With imperforate hymen, the hymen bulges. With absent vagina, the vaginal area is retracted upward and the hymen does not move. Vaginal septa may cause similar signs. The labia minora are prominent in the newborn, then atrophy, and are virtually absent until estrogens are produced at adolescence. Adhesions of the labia in older girls may be caused by infection, irritation, or local trauma, including abuse, and may cause dysuria.

Figure 6-3
Inspection of the vagina using a vaginoscope for children and simple illumination with a flashlight.

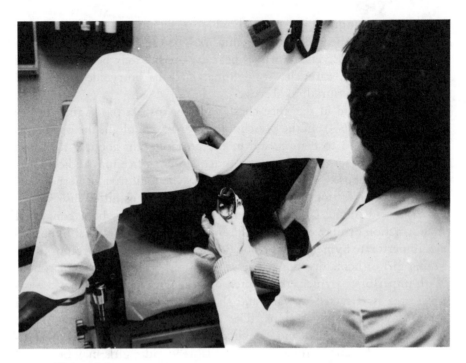

Figure 6-4
Proper draping for pelvic examination. *(From Scipien GM et al (editors): Comprehensive pediatric nursing, ed 3, New York, 1986, McGraw-Hill.)*

A bloody *vaginal discharge* is normal but not common up to the fourth week of life and at menarche. Vaginal bleeding in children less than 8 years old is usually attributable to foreign bodies, injury, or constitutional isosexual precocity; ovarian tumors, botryoid sarcoma, and carcinoma of the cervix may present similarly. A mucoid vaginal discharge is frequently noted. In the diaper age this usually results from irritation by the diaper or the powder used in the diaper region. In older children a foul discharge may be due to tight panties or pants, intertrigo, masturbation, pinworms, infection secondary to a foreign body, or allergy. A thin watery discharge is common in girls for 2 to 3 years before onset of menstruation. Redness of the perineum may be caused by irritation of physical or chemical agents such as bubble baths but may also signal a urinary tract infection.

A purulent discharge may be attributable to gonorrhea. Profuse, frothy, foul-smelling pruritic discharges may be due to *Trichomonas* organisms. White adherent discharge suggests *Candida* infection.

Foreign bodies are usually palpated by rectal examination. A white, practically odorless discharge has no significance. Discharge significant of disease is usually accompanied by red inflammation in the surrounding vaginal and urethral structures. Urethral caruncle or *prolapse* of the urethra may be noted.

Vaginal palpation is usually omitted until near puberty. Note vaginal discharge or foreign body, size of uterus, and presence of ovaries. The normal uterus measures 1 to 2 cm, and the ovaries measure 0.5 to 1.0 cm until puberty.

The decision to have another person in the room during a vaginal examination should be made by the patient. Answer succinctly any questions the patient raises. Inspect pubic hair, mons pubis, labia majora, labia minora, clitoris, urethral meatus, and vaginal introitus for presence, location, infestations, appearance, and discharge. A large clitoris (a glans wider than 10 mm) may be normal or an isolated physical finding; however, it may indicate adrenal hyperplasia or any of the conditions associated with precocious puberty. The clitoris may not develop in adolescent girls with hypopituitarism or gonadal dysgenesis. The external genitalia grow very little until adolescence starts. In early puberty a rectal examination and an examination with the girl on the examining table with the knees bent and the soles of the feet flat allows the patient to hold the labia apart. Show the equipment to be used and explain any expected pain or pressure. In the older child, use the lithotomy position with stirrups. Palpate the vaginal orifice before inserting the warmed speculum. Feel for enlarged glands, a sign of sexually transmitted infectious diseases. Do not lubricate the speculum before insertion, since this precludes obtaining cultures. Use a vaginoscope with a 1 × 11 cm blade. Insert the blade vertically, then turn horizontally; open slowly with most pressure posteriorly. Maneuver the speculum until the cervix is seen. Do not stretch the hymen. Regardless of findings, do not use terms such as uterus is *small, infantile,* or *underdeveloped,* since these may frighten the patient. The normal ratio of fundus to cervix is 1 to 3 in the infant, 1 to 1 in the pubertal girl, and 3 to 1 in the mature woman.

The cervix is normally pink and smooth, but columnar epithelium may extend over the junction, resembling erosion. The color becomes blue during pregnancy. Tenderness on moving the cervix or in the area of the fallopian tubes suggests pelvic inflammatory disease. An adnexal mass may be abscess, ectopic pregnancy, endometriosis, or ovarian cyst. An enlarged uterus occurs with intrauterine or ectopic pregnancy. Observe the vaginal wall for discharge or ulcers. Take cultures of any discharge, and endocervical swab for Papanicolaou (PAP) smear. Remove the speculum slowly. Proceed with bimanual examination. Cover the gloved index and middle fingers with sterile lubricant and press posteriorly. Note any firmness or masses in the vagina. Note if the cervix is firm or soft and if the os is open or closed. Palpate the uterus between the abdomen and vagina: note its size, shape, and position and whether it is soft, firm, smooth, or tender. Palpate the adnexa on either side for enlargement, tenderness, or masses. Ovaries are normally less than 1 cm in size before puberty and up to 3 cm in size at puberty and may not be palpable unless enlarged.

The average adolescent development in girls proceeds as follows: breast development after the age of 8, pubic hair at about the age of 12, increase in height velocity at the age of 12, and menarche and axillary hair before the age of 13.

In the male patient, make a note if the position of the urethral orifice is not at the tip of the glans. *Hypospadias* exists if the opening is on the ventral (inferior) surface, and *epispadias* is present if the opening is on the dorsal surface of the penis. The prepuce is examined for infection, posthitis, and *phimosis* (a small opening of the prepuce). Some adhesions of the prepuce to the glans are normal until about the age of 4. Foreign body may be felt as a hard mass in the urethra. The prepuce may be inflamed, swollen, and tender. Inflammation of the glans (balanitis) may cause urinary obstruction. Pink pearly papules (elongated papillae 1 to 3 mm in size on the corona of the penis) are normal in adolescents. Venereal warts are less uniform in size. Herpes simplex may resemble a small tender pimple, whereas a syphilitic chancre is a larger, less tender ulcer.

An enlarged penis may be noted in children with precocious puberty, central nervous system lesions, some testicular tumors, and adrenal hyperplasia. In congenital adrenal hyperplasia the penis is large but the testes are of normal size. The penis may appear small if it is obscured by fat in corpulent boys. The penis is small in adolescent boys with hypopituitarism.

Observe the *meatal* opening. Stenosis may cause the opening to appear round instead of slitlike. Ulcers may cause obstruction to urinary flow. Note strength of stream in both sexes; decreased stream indicates obstruction.

Next look at the *scrotum*. Normally the scrotum of a child who is not cold or frightened is loose and the testes and cords can be felt in it. Anything else in the scrotum is abnormal. If the scrotum appears large, suspect hernia or hydrocele or both. Often, especially in premature infants, the scrotal sac appears small, empty, and underdeveloped. Put your index finger and thumb together to make an inverted "V," place them about ½ inch above the center of the inguinal ligament, and gently push toward the scrotum. Somewhere along the inguinal canal, a soft mass will be felt. Then try to push this mass into the scrotum. Once in the scrotum, grasp the mass with the thumb and forefinger of the opposite hand. If it can be brought to this position even though it may immediately retract, the mass is a normally descended *testis*. Repeat the procedure on the opposite side. If the mass is palpable in the inguinal canal but cannot be pushed down or if the testis is not felt, suspect an undescended testis or abdominal testis. In the older child, one maneuver to bring the testis down is as follows: Have the boy sit in a chair with his heels on the seat, grabbing his knees. The extra abdominal pressure may push the testis into the scrotum. A small, flat, underdeveloped scrotum is probably the most accurate indication of true maldescent (cryptorchidism), usually resulting from defects in the inguinal canal but possibly signaling hypogonadism.

The testes are smooth and usually about 1 cm in size until puberty. At stage II of puberty, length is 2 to 3.2 cm; at stage III, 3.3 to 4.0 cm; at stage IV, 4.1 to 4.9 cm; and at stage V, 5 cm. They remain small in children with hypopituitarism. They are large in boys with fragile X syndrome and are uneven and enlarged with infection or tumor of the testis. They are large with precocious puberty but not with precocious puberty secondary to adrenal hyperplasia. Hard, enlarged testis without pain suggests tumor.

Average penile length is 4 cm at birth, 5 cm at 4 years of age, 6 cm at 11 years of age, and 12 cm at the end of adolescence. Micropenis is found in children with chromosomal abnormalities, Prader-Willi syndrome, and other dysmorphic syndromes. If the penis is normal or small and the testes are firm and small in the adolescent, gonadal dysgenesis (Klinefelter's syndrome) may be present. The left testis is usually lower than the right. The opposite may indicate complete situs inversus.

If the scrotum appears large, changes size, or enlarges with coughing or crying, place one finger on the external ring and palpate the scrotum. If the mass in the scrotum feels firm, it is probably normal testis. If something is palpated in addition to the testis and cord, try to determine whether the sensation obtained is that of fluid, gas, or solid structure. Try to reduce the mass in the scrotum by pushing the contents back through the external ring. Masses that cannot be reduced include incarcerated hernia hydrocele, varicocele, and spermatocele, in addition to normal structures.

Fluid in the scrotum usually indicates the presence of a *hydrocele*. Hydroceles are found frequently in children under 2 years of age, are usually not tender, and with closed tunica vaginalis testis, usually do not change size when reduction is attempted. Fluid fluctuating in volume denotes the presence of a patent tunica vaginalis testis or indirect inguinal hernia. Varicocele feels like a "bag of worms" because of the dilation of the pampiniform veins and usually occurs on the left. Spermatocele is a benign cyst on the head of the epididymis.

Next, shine a light through the mass. If the mass (except the testis) transilluminates and is irreducible, fluid is probably present. If the mass does not transilluminate and is irreducible, hernia is probably present. The use of transillumination in young children may be misleading because bowel in a hernial sac may transilluminate.

If a bulge occurs in the inguinal canal, a mass that is neither testis nor fluid is found in the scrotum, or you get the sensation of gas (crepitus) on palpation, the patient has a visible *hernia*. If you feel crepitus when you try to push the mass through the external ring, hernia is also indicated. Tenderness may be noted. In contrast to hydroceles, hernias are usually tender. Next, auscultate over the scrotal sac. Peristaltic sounds help to indicate the presence of a hernia.

Hernias that cannot be reduced in spite of careful manipulation are said to be *incarcerated*. Hernias that feel swollen or have become gangrenous are *strangulated* from the tight constriction of the neck of the sac.

Finally, if a hernia or hydrocele is suspected, feel over the internal ring with the flat part of the index finger and roll the spermatic cord beneath the fingers as it lies in the inguinal canal. Though the ring is normally open, only a thin 1 to 2 mm solid structure should be felt going through the ring. If the cord feels thickened or like silk being rubbed on silk, peritoneum is going through the ring, denoting a hernia that may be invisible. The size of the structures in the canal can also be determined in this manner, and thickened structures may indicate polyarteritis or another abnormality. Occasionally a hydrocele of the spermatic cord can be felt and may be mistaken for an incarcerated hernia. Careful palpation of the mass helps to separate the upper end of the hydrocele from the internal ring, which is not possible with a hernia.

If the infant's mother reports the presence of a hernia but none is found, the following maneuvers may make the hernia obvious: Stand the infant on the examining table and place the flat of your hand on the abdomen. Pump the abdomen in and out with several short frequent strokes, and the hernial sac will become apparent. The older child may sit on a stool and hold the knees while you try to straighten the legs. The hernial sac will then fill.

Acute *swelling* of the scrotum with discoloration may result from torsion of the spermatic cord, a surgical emergency. Acute painful swelling also occurs in boys with orchitis, epididymitis, or rarely, torsion of the testis appendages. With torsion the testicle is higher in the scrotum than it should be and may appear to lie transversely. With epididymitis the testicle is in the normal position, and the long axis usually is in the axis of the body. The spermatic cord is tender and swollen with epididymitis and tender but not swollen with torsion. Elevation of the swollen tender mass increases the pain in epididymitis. Epididymitis is usually caused by infection and accompanied by signs of urethral infection, but it may be a presenting sign of sarcoid. The testis may be dislocated into the inguinal canal after trauma.

Differential diagnosis of testicular torsion, incarcerated inguinal hernia, epididymitis, and orchitis—all of which cause scrotal swelling— may be difficult. With testicular torsion the spermatic artery on the involved side does not pulsate. Pulsation is increased with orchitis, epididymitis, and torsion of the testicular appendix. Orchitis is usually accompanied by mumps or other viral infection.

The *cremasteric reflex* is tested by stroking the inner aspect of the thigh. The testis will rise in the scrotum, sometimes going up into the canal. This reflex is normal at any age. Absence may indicate a low spinal cord lesion, as in poliomyelitis, but it is also frequently absent in normal boys, especially under the age of 6 months and over the age of 12 years.

Examine the *lymph nodes* in the inguinal region for size and tenderness. Ordinarily three or four 0.5 to 1.0 cm glands are not abnormal. Tenderness or enlargement always indicates infection or any of the systemic diseases associated with generalized enlarged nodes.

The average adolescent development in boys proceeds as follows: testicular enlargement, 11.5 years of age; pubic hair, 12.5 years of age; increase in height velocity, 14 years of age; and facial and axillary hair, 14.5 years of age.

ANUS AND RECTUM

Examine the anal region regularly in infants and children. However, rectal examination is not performed in a routine examination but is reserved for those children with symptoms referable to the lower gastrointestinal tract or those with abdominal pain.

Note the *buttocks* for masses and firmness. Masses over the coccygeal area are usually sacrococcygeal tumors. Tufts of hair, meningocele, pilonidal dimple, and perianal abscess may be noted easily in this area. If a pilonidal dimple is present, carefully inspect it for presence of a sinus.

Abscesses may be caused by *rectal fistula*. Therefore, determine the extent of any rectal fistula by observation, and probe if the full extent of the fistula cannot be visualized.

The buttocks are usually firm, even in advanced malnutrition; however, in cystic fibrosis and celiac syndrome, they are flattened. The skin creases of the buttocks are usually asymmetric but may indicate the presence of congenitally dislocated hips. Skin creases of the buttocks are especially prominent in children with recent weight loss.

Anal fissure appears as a cut or tear in the mucosa. It is one of the most frequent causes of constipation or rectal bleeding in an infant up to the age of 2, and many cause infantile "colic." Anal fissure is best noted by placing the infant on the abdomen, pulling the buttocks apart, and noting the fissure and asymmetry of mucosal folds. Bleeding may occur following this maneuver.

Note prolapse of the rectal mucosa. It may be a cause of infantile colic. It may be caused by chronic constipation, straining, or diarrhea and may occur with cystic fibrosis or neurologic or anatomic abnormalities. It is rarely seen in pertussis.

Note other *protrusions* from the anus. Small mucosal tabs have no significance; however, cherry-red, round protrusions may be rectal polyps and cause rectal bleeding. Solid dark protrusions are hemorrhoids and may be caused by portal hypertension. They are rarely found in children. Large flat tabs of the skin may be condylomas, a sign of papilloma virus infection, syphilis, or sexual abuse.

Occasionally pinworms are noted in the perianal area in the folds of rectal mucosa; these may cause rectal itching. A dark *ring* around the rectal mucosa may be an early sign of lead poisoning.

Most of the eruptions around the rectum in the young result from diaper rash. Usually the eruption is a generalized reddened or brawny area with vesicles or papules. However, pustules may be present and represent secondary infection of the diaper rash or perianal cellulitis resulting from streptococcus.

A *rectal* examination is best done with the infant or child lying supine with the legs flexed. If the child is old enough, ask the child to empty the bladder before this examination. Ordinarily, your fifth finger is long enough to give the required information in the infant and hurts the patient less than a larger finger. Because you may have better control and mobility of the index finger, use it for more precise information. Grease the anus and finger cot well before insertion. Imperforate anus is noted immediately, since the finger cannot enter beyond the dimple.

Note sphincter *tone*. A patulous rectum is associated with sexual abuse or a low cord injury, including myelomeningocele and diastematomyelia. A tight sphincter is generally a developmental variation indicating stenosis. Anal stenosis may cause constipation and pain on defecation. Rectovaginal *fistulas* are noted by having the finger enter the vagina through the rectum.

Occasionally you will feel a shelflike protuberance 2 to 5 cm above the anus. This feeling with absence of feces in the rectum may be a sign of aganglionic megacolon. Anterior position of the anal opening with a posterior shelf on rectal examination is a sign of anterior ectopic anus, a cause of chronic constipation. If position is uncertain, measure in girls from fourchette to anus to coccyx and in boys from the base of the scrotum. The distance of fourchette or scrotum to anus divided by fourchette or scrotum to coccyx is 0.39 or 0.56, respectively. Marked deviation indicates displacement.

The anus and rectum may be distended with feces in children with mental delay, chronic constipation, or psychogenic difficulties. Absence of feces in the rectum in an acutely ill child may indicate ileus, peritonitis, or obstruction.

Note masses. Fecal masses of any consistency can be removed. A tender mass in the lower quadrants may be found with a low intussusception. A right lower quadrant mass is occasionally noted with acute appendicitis or appendiceal abscess and sometimes with regional ileitis. Polyps may occasionally be felt in the rectum. Masses that displace the rectum forward frequently are teratomas. Other masses described under examination of the abdomen are also noted and have similar significance.

Occasionally a *prostate* will be palpated as a flat mass several centimeters up and on the midline anterior wall of the rectum. Any prostate felt larger than 1 cm in size before the age of 10 may indicate precocious puberty or congenital adrenal hyperplasia. After puberty the prostate is 2 to 3 cm in size and smooth. A tender prostate indicates infection; an uneven or large prostate suggests tumor.

Rectal examination is also useful in palpating the *uterus*. In the pubertal child and occasionally in younger children, the ovaries may also be palpated. The prepubertal uterus is felt as a 1 to 2 cm oval mass anterior to the rectum and about 3 or 4 cm above the symphysis pubis. When the ovaries are palpable before puberty, they are about 0.5 to 1.0 cm in diameter, about 2 to 3 cm laterad and just above the uterus. Foreign bodies in the vagina or rectum can also be felt by this method.

Even though this examination is usually uncomfortable and reserved for the last part of the physical, a rectal examination can frequently localize tenderness in the abdomen. After your finger is well up in the rectum, place it in the midline and press the other hand toward the finger. Note facial expression. Next, move the finger and the abdominal hand to the left, and repeat on the right. Differences in facial expression or rigidity of the lower abdomen are clues to abdominal or rectal pathology.

Sensation should be tested in children who are suspected of having a spinal cord lesion or a patulous rectal sphincter. Use a pin to touch the perineal region at closely approximated points. Twitching of the perineum normally occurs with a slight lateral movement of the anus. Absence of this reflex suggests lower motor neuron lesion.

If you want to visualize the rectal mucosa for suspected internal rectal fissure, polyp, hemorrhoid, colitis, proctitis, or bleeding site, the examination may be done with relative ease with a small proctoscope or without special equipment. Grease a clean test tube and push it about 5 cm into the rectum. Place a small light just behind your shoulder, shining into the tube. Slowly withdraw the tube, and note the mucosa as it falls back into place.

7

EXTREMITIES, JOINTS, SPINE, AND MUSCLES

I N PRACTICE, THE physician usually examines the bones, joints, and muscles simultaneously. Then, if abnormalities are found, the systems under suspicion are examined individually.

The order of examination of these systems depends largely on the age, condition, and cooperation of the child. If the child walks, preliminary observations of posture, gait, and stance can be made immediately. The position the child assumes during the examination may be noted either during this part of the examination or as part of the general appearance of the patient.

EXTREMITIES

In the 2- to 6-year-old age group, you may begin the physical examination with observations of the hands and feet. Most children of these ages are happy to show their hands and feet when requested and are especially happy to see no instruments present at the beginning of the examination. Persistently pink hands and feet are a sign of poor nutrition, poor hygiene, or other types of deprivation.

Infants who hold both their arms immobile in 90-degree flexion at the elbow when lying, sitting, or standing may be suffering from emotional deprivation. Those infants appearing to look at one arm for a long time or who hold one arm in an unusual position for 1 or 2 minutes may have infantile autism. Such posturing is normal up to about 6 months of age. Stereotypic hand movements and hand wringing in young girls may be a sign of Rett syndrome.

Note congenital *anomalies* of the arms, hands, legs, and feet. These include amelia (absence of the part), webbing, and extra digits.

Length and shape of the extremities are usually determined by nutritional and congenital factors. Abnormalities (for example, long, thin extremities) are noted in children with arachnodactyly. Broad, short extremities are noted in children with Down syndrome, mucopolysaccharidoses, or chondrodystrophies. Apparent shortening of the thumb and fourth and fifth fingers occurs almost always in children with pseudohypoparathyroidism.

Shortening of an extremity is usually congenital but may result from diseases of the epiphyses or cerebral palsy. Inequality of leg length may be present in children after femoral fractures or with dislocation of the hip or other hip disorders.

Lengthening of an extremity is usually congenital but may result from large hemangiomas, lymphangiomas, arteriovenous fistula, neurofibromatosis, or hemihypertrophy. Generalized enlargement of the extremities may occur from any of these factors and, when unilateral, may cause hemigigantism. Enlargement may also be attributable to lymphedema praecox or congenital lymphedema (Milroy's disease) as a manifestation of ovarian dysgenesis, Turner's syndrome, or edema.

Inspect fingers and toes for *clubbing*. Elevation of the nail base is an early sign of clubbing. Later, the entire end of the finger, including the nail region, seems expanded and rounded when compared with the remainder of the finger. Ask the child to oppose both thumbnails. Normally a small diamond-shaped opening is visible. With clubbing, no space is present. Clubbing may occur in any condition of reduced circulating oxygen, such as cyanotic congenital heart disease or chronic pulmonary disease, and also in patients with chronic liver disease or bacterial endocarditis. Clubbing may be a presenting sign of cystic fibrosis, Crohn's disease, ulcerative colitis, celiac disease, gastroesophageal reflux, intestinal parasite infestation, and thalassemia.

Pain and *tenderness* in the extremities are usually caused by trauma or infection. Pain, especially of the legs, is noted in infants with scurvy. Infants under 3 months of age with congenital syphilis may have pain causing pseudoparalyses. Tenderness over the sartorius muscle may be noted in children with tuberculous meningitis. Tenderness elicited at a point in the bone by sharp percussion of the distal end of the bone suggests the presence of osteomyelitis (Figure 7-1). Inability to supinate the hand with the arm held in flexion and pain in the elbow indicate subluxation of the head of the radius.

Pain in the knee or foot may result from local disease, but it also requires examination of the hips. Pain in the knee increased with internal rotation of the tibia may be caused by osteochondritis dissecans. Pain in a

Figure 7-1
Striking the foot to elicit pain of osteomyelitis in the tibia or fibula.

bone, worse at night and rapidly relieved by aspirin, is characteristic of osteoid osteoma.

Note the *temperature* of the extremities, taking special care to note whether the temperature bilaterally is equal. Differences in temperature are usually attributed to neurologic or vascular abnormalities. Cold, pallid extremities may occur after sympathetic nervous system stimulation or may be a manifestation of venous or arterial thrombosis or embolism. With nervous system lesions, pulsations are usually present, whereas with vascular lesions, pulsations are usually diminished or absent.

Necrosis of the extremity, or *gangrene,* may result from obliteration of the vascular supply. The area is cold, avascular, pallid, and tender, with loss of muscle power. The area may gradually become black and less painful as necrosis proceeds. It may ooze and be moist and obviously infected, or it may be dry. It may occur in infants after embolism, particularly from the umbilical venous system, after severe trauma or infection to the part, and sometimes after frostbite.

Enlargement of the bones may be caused by infection in the bone. Swelling with joint tenderness, heat, and redness near but not in the joint is characteristic of osteomyelitis. Swelling may result from periosteal hemorrhage, as in scurvy; from cortical thickening, as in congenital syphilis, vitamin A poisoning, or infantile cortical hyperostosis; from localized increased calcification, as in callus formation after fracture or in rickets; or from bone cysts or tumors. Auscultation over the area of the swelling may reveal a bruit, more common in osteomyelitis than in the other causes of increased vascularity of the bone.

Enlargement of the tibial tubercles with tenderness is characteristic of Osgood-Schlatter disease, probably from stress on the patellar tendon.

Bony, painless swelling at the epiphysis adjacent to the knee or wrist joints is one of the most definite signs of rickets. Symmetric swelling of both hands or both feet in infants may indicate the hand-foot syndrome of sickle cell anemia.

Other *deformities* of the bones are usually caused by fractures. Fractures are noted by the patient's inability to use the limb, by deformity, or by excess motion in the bone with pain and crepitation. Auscultation at the proximal epiphysis while tapping the distal end of a bone causes a difference in sound on the fractured side from the sound elicited on the nonfractured side. Fractures are almost always caused by trauma and may suggest child abuse. Multiple fractures may result from polyostotic fibrous dysplasia, bone cysts, other diseases of the parathyroid gland, prolonged bed rest, or osteogenesis imperfecta.

Note *shape* of the bones. Lateral bowing of the tibia (genu varum) is present when the child stands with the medial malleoli in apposition, and a persistent space of more than 2 cm is observed between the medial surfaces of the knees. Frequently the infant is bowlegged for 1 year after starting to walk. Significant genu varum may result from anomalies of the feet or from rickets. Anterior curvature of the tibia may indicate congenital syphilis. Excess bowing just below the knee may indicate osteochondrosis deformans, Blount's disease, or tibia vara.

Knock-knees (genu valgum) can be determined when, with the knees together, the medial malleoli persistently are separated more than 2 cm. Knock-knees are usually normal in children from about 2 to 3½ years of age. Knock-knees may also be seen in children with pronated feet, rickets, or syphilis.

Bony hard enlargement of the medial or external aspects of the femoral or tibial epiphyses is usually a normal variant but may occur with rickets, other metabolic bone diseases, or with dysgenesis of the knees such as dysplasia epiphysialis hemimelia.

Tibial torsion, a twisting of the tibia probably initiated by the intrauterine position, is best determined with the patient on the back and the knees facing upward. Both the forefoot and the hindfoot will be held in a plane but not in line with the knees. With the tibial tubercle and the patella in a straight line, place your fingers on the malleoli. In an infant the line joining the four malleoli should be parallel to the table. In the older child, up to 20-degree external torsion is normal. With any greater deviation or if the lateral malleolus is anterior to the medial malleolus, inward tibial torsion may be present. With fixed deformities of the foot such as metatarsus varus the forefoot will be adducted in this position, but the hindfoot will be in a straight line with the patella.

Note the *feet* for abnormalities. The feet at birth are usually held in varus or valgus attitude, almost never straight. An easy method to determine whether this position, which was the intrauterine position, will straighten is simply to scratch first the outside and then the inside of the lower border of the foot. In self-correctable deformities the foot will assume a right angle with the leg. More severe anomalies, such as clubfeet or metatarsus varus, either can be straightened only with forceful manual stretching or cannot be straightened by manual means at all (Figure 7-2).

Because all children have a fat pad under the arch, the feet may appear flat until the child has walked for 2 years. A very high-arched foot (pes cavus) may be noted in some normal children or may be seen in patients with Friedreich's ataxia, poliomyelitis, or various lower motor neuron lesions. Talipes equinus, with short heel cords and weight-bearing on the toes, may be a characteristic of cerebral palsy or muscular diseases; it results in spasm and contracture of the muscles of the leg and may

Figure 7-2
A, Forefoot adduction; heel inversion. **B,** Talipes equinovarus.

cause "toe walking." Many normal children walk on their toes until the age of 3.

Toe walking may also indicate muscle imbalance, spasticity, muscular dystrophy of the Duchenne type, or disorders causing weakness of the peroneal and anterior tibial muscles. Children with septic arthritis of the hip walk on their toes to relieve strain around the hip. Some autistic and some normal children also toe walk.

Examine the heel cords with the patient in the supine position and the knee extended. Grasp the foot by the heel (Figure 7-3), with the sole lying in your hand; slightly invert the foot to lock the heel and then dorsiflex it. Tight cords are present if dorsiflexion cannot be carried to about 20 to 30 degrees beyond a right angle.

Note pronation of the feet. Pronation becomes apparent when the child stands. A pronated foot is flexible and may appear normal when the child lies on the table, but it will abduct at the forefoot when the patient stands, with obliteration of the long arch, bulging of the medial border of

Figure 7-3
Lock heel in palm of hand before testing for tight heel cords.

the foot, and outward angulation of the forefoot on the hindfoot. The medial malleolus may appear closer to the floor than normal, there may be knock-knees, and the thighs may appear adducted. The weight-bearing line, which is the line through the middle of the patella perpendicular to the floor, will cross the inner border of the foot instead of going through the second toe as is normal. From the back, the heel cord, which normally descends perpendicularly, will be noted to curve outward with eversion of the heel (valgus heel).

After examining the feet, look at the patient's shoes. Abnormal wear or misshapened shoes may help you to diagnose gait or foot disorders. Then note the patient's *gait* and *stance*. Observation in a room with a mirror at one end is helpful when studying the child's gait. Observe the anterior and posterior aspects simultaneously as the child walks toward and away from the mirror. The child should be wearing shoes or at least socks because bare feet on a cold floor may distort the gait.

Normally the 1- to 2-year-old child walks with a broadbased gait, frequently with the hands out to the side. Gradually as the child reaches the age of 3 or 4, the legs are brought together and the toes are straight ahead. The older child with a broadbased gait may have abnormal mechanics of the legs or feet, or the child may use this gait for balance if normal neural positioning and balancing mechanisms are defective. Watch for truncal ataxia as the child turns. Ask children over the age of 3 to walk on their toes to demonstrate distal muscle weakness, a sign of peripheral neuropathy. Ask children over the age of 4 to walk on their heels. Asymmetry suggests mild hemiparesis or hemiplegia. Ask children over the age of 5 to walk a line, heel to toe. Failure suggests a midline cerebellar lesion, a cerebellar tract defect, or gross motor incoordination.

Balance, at rest or while walking, is maintained by normal cerebellar function; normal vestibular nerve function; and good muscle, bone, and joint functions. Loss of balance may be attributed to cerebellar or vestibular disease or muscle weakness. Deviation to one side during walking may indicate cerebellar disease of that side. Lack of normal swing of the arm of that side suggests cerebellar involvement.

Toeing in (pigeon-toe) or toeing out may be noted. Children with pronated feet may toe in or toe out. Other orthopedic conditions causing toeing in include internal rotation of the hips, tibial torsion, and metatarsus adductus.

A scissors gait with a stiff crossing over of the legs as the child walks is noted, especially in children with a spastic type of cerebral palsy or with other types of mental delay. You can elicit this type of gait even in 7-month-old children if they are made to walk by gripping under the shoulders and pushing them along (Figure 7-4). A waddling gait may be noted in patients with bilateral dislocation of the hip or with coxa vara.

Note a *limp* of any type (see box). A limp may result from local infection; muscle, nerve, bone, or joint disease; or pain, but it is most commonly caused by trauma, fatigue, or a pathologic condition of the hip. Pain in the foot, ankle, knee, hip, or spine requires careful examination of all five areas because pathologic conditions of the hip or spine may be referred to the foot or knee. Children with intraabdominal inflammatory disease (for example, appendicitis, abscess, and retroperitoneal fibrosis) may limp.

You can examine the small child with a limp while the patient sits in the parent's lap. Observe the back, hips, buttocks, and extremities. Com-

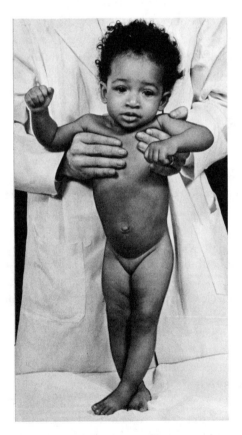

Figure 7-4
Scissors gait can be demonstrated before child can walk by grasping under axillae and pushing patient forward.

CAUSES OF LIMPING IN CHILDREN

Skeletal system

Trauma
Foreign body
Fracture
Infections
Postinfections

Joints

Synovitis
Arthralgia
Arthritis: rheumatoid, Kawasaki,
    Lyme
Sepsis
Dislocated hip
Slipped capital femoral epiphysis
Collagen vascular disease
Henoch-Schönlein purpura
Legg-Calvé-Perthes disease, aseptic
    necrosis
Toxins
Urticaria
Foot injuries
Bursitis

Nervous system

Neuropathic conditions

Spinal conditions

Spondylitis
Diskitis
Epidural abscess

Muscular system

Strain
Sprain
Myositis
Myopathic conditions

**Hemotologic and oncologic
    conditions**

Sickle cell disease
Leukemia
Neoplasms
Hemophilia
Serum sickness

Intraabdominal conditions

Appendicitis
Infection
Inflammatory bowel disease
Ovarian tumors, torsion
Pelvic inflammatory disease

pare the gluteal folds; look for asymmetry, swelling, and erythema of the two sides. Palpate for induration; warmth; tenderness over bones; muscle spasm; and effusion or distention of the joint capsules of the hip, knee, and ankle. Test each joint for motion, examining the suspect limb or joint last. Note restriction of flexion, extension, abduction, adduction, and rotation. Measure limb girth and length. Perform rectal and neurologic examinations.

Limp occurs with soft tissue injury anywhere in the lower extremity. Soft tissue injuries include *sprains* and *strains*. Abnormal laxity of a ligament after injury associated with local pain is characteristic of sprain. Swelling occurs because of bleeding into the joint. Disruption of a muscle-tendon unit is a strain. Similar signs may occur with epiphyseal fractures and dislocation of the patella. Foreign bodies, myositis, cellulitis, hives, bruising, and other lesions in the soft tissue may cause a limp.

Note *ataxia* as gross incoordination. Brain tumors, especially of the cerebellum, and encephalitides may be accompanied by ataxia. Ataxia caused by sensory or proprioceptive loss is worse with the eyes closed. The general weakness characteristic of the amyotonias or spasm of the muscles of the thigh in hip disease (p. 159) is sometimes mistaken for ataxia. Other cerebellar injuries, such as cerebral palsy with cerebellar involvement, the degenerative ataxias, some CNS infections, or tick paralysis, are especially likely to be followed by ataxia. Ataxia worsened by heat occurs with multiple sclerosis. Ataxia may occur as nonepileptiform seizures. A variety of drugs, including phenytoin, phenobarbital, and the antihistamines, may cause ataxia in sensitive persons. Vestibular damage, as is sometimes seen in children treated with streptomycin, may be followed by ataxia. For the teenage athlete, a short examination is helpful (Table 7-1).

JOINTS

Examine the joints for *heat,* tenderness, *swelling, effusion, redness,* and *limitation* or pain on motion. Redness, heat, and tenderness—signs of infection—are noted by observation and palpation. Effusion in the joint, a sign of any type of joint irritation, can be best determined by ballottement of the joint or by tapping on one side of the joint and feeling protrusion on the other side as a fluid wave is elicited. In children the most common cause of tenderness in one joint with limitation of motion but without other physical signs is synovitis of traumatic or nonspecific origin.

With the joint extended, try to push fluid from the outer to the medial side of the joint with the flat part of your hand. A bulge of the synovial lining, particularly on the medial side of the knee previously described, indicates effusion. Transillumination helps recognize the presence of fluid.

Swollen, hot joints are seen in children with rheumatoid arthritis; rheumatic fever; Lyme disease; allergic, toxic, and infectious arthritis; serum sickness; hemarthrosis; or osteochondritis. Motion is limited in these conditions, usually because of pain and spasm of the overlying muscles and tendons. Arthritis of rheumatic fever is painful without much swelling and responds to aspirin more rapidly than rheumatoid arthritis in which the joints are stiff. In rheumatic fever and systemic lupus erythematosus the swelling may be reducible (Jaccoud's syndrome). Swelling,

TABLE 7-1

The 2-minute orthopedic examination

Instructions	Observation
Stand facing examiner	Acromioclavicular joints, general habitus
Look at ceiling, floor, over both shoulders	Cervical spine motion
Shrug shoulders (examiner resists)	Trapezius strength
Abduct shoulders 90 degrees (examiner resists at 90 degrees)	Deltoid strength
Full external rotation of arms	Shoulder motion
Flex and extend elbows	Elbow motion
Arms at sides, elbows 90 degrees flexed; pronate and supinate wrists	Elbow and wrist motion
Spread fingers; make fist	Hand or finger motion and deformities
Tighten (contract) quadriceps; relax quadriceps	Symmetry and knee effusion; ankle effusion
"Duck walk" four steps (away from examiner with buttocks on heels)	Hip, knee, and ankle motion
Turn back to examiner	Shoulder symmetry, scoliosis
Keep knees straight, touch toes	Scoliosis, hip motion, hamstring tightness
Raise up on toes, raise heels	Calf symmetry, leg strength

Reproduced from Sports Medicine: Health care for young athletes, 1983, Elk Grove, Ill, AAP.

pain, and limited motion in the knee after injury may be caused by a dislocated patella. Pain in the joint without physical findings is arthralgia and may be caused by any condition discussed previously or by strains, overactivity, allergic reactions, Kawasaki disease, or human immunodeficiency or other viral diseases and is vaguely specific.

Limitation of joint motion without pain may occur as a congenital malformation. Flexion deformities of the fingers and toes are common. Children with multiple congenital dislocations, as in arthrogryposis, may have severe flexion deformities of many joints. Limitation of joint motion is also common in children with various spastic neurologic disorders, which are described in Chapter 8.

Detect excess joint motion by hyperflexing or hyperextending the joint. It usually results from relaxation of the structures surrounding the joint but is exaggerated in children with Down syndrome, general debility, amyotonia congenita, and Ehlers-Danlos syndrome. Hypermobility of the joints, especially the wrists, is seen in most children with chorea because of poor muscle tone and in children with rickets or malnutrition. Hyperextension of the knees (genu recurvatum) may be attributed to the intrauterine position, or it may be noted in children with spina bifida, arthrogryposis, agenesis of the patella, or other malformations.

In infants, investigate the *hips* routinely for congenital dislocation or subluxation. With the infant on the back, flex the legs at the knees and attempt internal and external *rotation* by holding the knees and simultaneously rotating the thighs (Figures 7-5 and 7-6). It is thus easy to see whether the rotation is equal on both sides. Unequal rotation is usually caused by decreased mobility of one joint. The hips can be abducted and externally rotated so that the knees touch the tabletop in most infants. With unilateral subluxation, abduction is limited on the affected side (Figure 7-6). A "click" may either be normal or a sign of dislocation after this maneuver. Grasp the outer aspect of one thigh with the middle finger over the greater trochanter. Lift and abduct the thigh. A "clunk" indicates that a dislocated hip has been reduced (Ortolani's click).

Determine *piston mobility* in children with hip joint dislocations by holding the hip region with one hand, grasping the thigh with the other hand, and pulling the hands apart gently (Figure 7-7). Motion that occurs in a Slinky toy is piston mobility. A little motion, perhaps up to 1 cm, is normally present, but with congenital dislocation the hip motion may

Figure 7-5
Internal rotation of the hips.

Figure 7-6
External rotation of the hips. Note that angles made by each leg are
equal.

Figure 7-7
Piston mobility. Grasp thigh firmly.

have a range from 2 cm above to 2 cm below the socket. As the child gets
older, tightness of the adductor muscles is noted, and the *gluteal folds* may
be uneven. Uneven gluteal folds may be seen in normal children.

In addition to recognized congenital dislocation, progressive subluxation of the hip occurs in older children, especially in those who are
obese. The child with dislocation of the hip usually has a painless limp

with apparent shortening of the leg on the involved side. When the child is asked to stand on the normal limb and raise the other leg, the pelvis on the involved side rises to maintain balance. When the patient is asked to stand on the leg with the dislocated hip and raise the normal limb, the abductor muscles cannot raise the pelvis and it drops (Trendelenburg's sign) (Figure 7-8). A painless limp, worse with fatigue, occurs also with coxa plana, especially in boys.

A painful limp with limited motion, especially in the morning, is usually seen in children with tuberculosis of the hip. In addition, in this disease the hip is first abducted and later adducted with flexion on the pelvis. If it appears that children are simulating limps or abnormal gaits, tell them to run, touch a spot, and return. Usually they will concentrate on

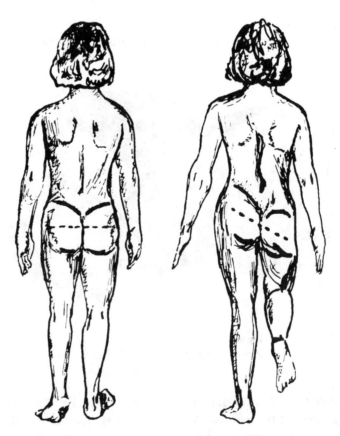

Figure 7-8
Trendelenburg's sign. When standing on both feet, pelvis is level; when standing on affected side, normal side drops.

your instructions and forget to simulate. Limited flexion or extension of the knee with a limp may result from dislocation or chondromalacia of the patella (peripatellar bursitis) after injury, osteochondritis, other bone disease, or all other joint diseases.

Limited motion of the *elbow* with weakness after injury suggests tennis elbow. Pain is over the lateral epicondyle because of strain. In the child under the age of 2, inability to supinate the hand with the arm held in flexion, along with pain in the elbow, indicates subluxation of the head of the radius.

Knee injuries

Examine the unaffected knee first. Inspect when the patient is in the supine position, sitting, and standing. Note angular deformities, the presence of effusion, ecchymoses, abrasions, scars, and gait if weight-bearing is possible. Check for muscle atrophy of the thigh or calf. Check range of motion last if effusion is present. If effusion occurs shortly after injury, suspect a serious injury with hemarthrosis. Delayed onset of effusion after injury suggests strains or an inflammatory process.

Palpate to identify the site of maximum pain. Pain in the joint suggests a cartilage or ligament injury. Stress the joint by abducting and adducting with the patient in the supine position and with 30-degree flexion. Pain with the patient in the supine position suggests medial ligament injury; at 30 degrees, it indicates collateral ligament.

Test with 90-degree flexion, pulling on the proximal tibia. Excess displacement indicates cruciate ligament tears.

Flex the hip and knee and rotate the foot. A click indicates a torn miniscus. Locking of the knee suggests intraarticular loose bodies. Pain in the tibial tubercle suggests Osgood-Schlatter disease resulting from bursitis or fracture. Pain or dislocation of the patella may indicate fracture. If the patella is not palpable, suspect peripatellar bursitis.

Shoulder injuries

Compare both shoulders. Asymmetry may result from edema, deformity, trauma, septic arthritis, or osteomyelitis. Squaring of the shoulder suggests dislocation. Prominence of the distal clavicle may be attributed to acromioclavicular separation. A double bulge on the anterior surface of the upper arm when the elbow is flexed suggests rupture of the biceps tendon. Note the point of maximum tenderness and try to identify the part of the joint, tendon, muscle, or bone involved. Have the child fully abduct the arm to locate limitation.

SPINE

Examine the spine in routine physical examinations. Observe the infant in the supine position. The patient may kick and move during the examination. Then place the infant on the abdomen. In the older child, make observations with the patient in the sitting or standing position. Note the way the child stands or walks.

Tufts of hair, dimples, hemangiomas, discolorations, cysts, and masses are frequently seen near the spine. These may cause tethering of the cord. A tuft of hair over a small dimple in the midline usually indicates the presence of an underlying spina bifida, or it may simply be an ectodermal anomaly. Spina bifida occulta can occasionally be determined by pressing carefully over the area under suspicion when the trunk is flexed. The spinous processes above and below the spina bifida will feel thin and well formed, whereas the spinous process of the defective vertebra may feel split.

A small dimple in the midline anywhere from the coccyx to the skull usually indicates a dermoid sinus. These dimples are important to record as possible entry points of infection to the CNS.

Palpate and transilluminate *masses* over the spine. Nontender masses of varied color and consistency with a thin covering are usually meningoceles. Meningoceles, which communicate with the CNS, can usually be distinguished from noncommunicating masses by palpation. If signs of increased intracranial pressure such as bulging of the fontanel occur, it is likely that the contents of the mass communicate with the spinal canal. Cystic masses that transilluminate may be teratoma, meningocele, or lipomeningocele. Nontender, noncommunicating masses near the spine are usually lipomas or fibromas. Soft masses feeling like lipomas, usually with skin dimples, may also extend into the CNS and are lipomeningoceles.

Tender masses not communicating with the spinal canal are usually infectious and include tuberculous spondylitis and tuberculous and perinephric abscesses. Deep tenderness over the spine is usually caused by trauma of the spine or surrounding structures. Localized spine tenderness is best elicited by punching with the side of your hand or by tapping with the reflex hammer. Localized tenderness may indicate a cord tumor or injury or infection of an intervertebral disk (diskitis). Masses covered by skin over the sacrum or coccyx may be teratomas. These are firm and can usually also be felt on rectal examination.

Examine the spine for intrinsic *motion*. Limitation of flexion is easily demonstrated by asking patients to sit up from a prone position. They will turn over and maintain the position of the back with pokerlike rigidity. If patients are sitting, ask them to kiss their knees to demonstrate limitation of forward bending. If you place your fingers on several of the patients' adjoining spinous processes, normally they will move separately as patients bend the trunk laterally. With stiffness of the spine, your fingers move as a unit.

The spine is stiff in children with CNS infections, especially meningitis or tetanus; with diseases or anomalies of the bones such as osteomyelitis of the spine, epiphysitis of the vertebrae, or hemivertebrae; or with adjacent lesions such as peritonitis or perinephric abscesses. Occasionally with severe trauma to the back, the spine will be rigid. Causes of limitation of motion of the spine in adults, such as osteoarthritis, protruding intervertebral disk, and lumbosacral strain, occur infrequently in adolescents. Severe pain and tenderness over the spine, particularly at night, may result from a tuberculous abscess or cord tumor. Inflammatory disease or a tumor of or near the spine may cause referred pain to the abdomen, hips, knees, or legs.

Limitation of motion of the neck by muscle spasm is a prime neurologic sign of nervous system disease and is discussed with other lesions of the neck. Nonneurologic causes of limitation of motion of the neck include rheumatoid arthritis of the cervical vertebrae; adjacent infections such as cervical adenitis and retropharyngeal abscess; rotatory subluxation of the cervical vertebrae; fracture or congenital anomalies of the vertebrae, especially hemivertebrae; or shortening of the sternocleidomastoid muscle producing torticollis (wryneck).

Opisthotonos, or hyperextension of the spine, is noted periodically in all normal infants or in infants with breath-holding spells. Recurrent hyperextension to lessen obstruction from tracheal compression strongly suggests vascular ring. True opisthotonos, which is a rigid, prolonged hyperextension of the spine, usually denotes a completely decerebrate individual and is observed in those with severe mental delay, kernicterus, or severe infections of the CNS. This condition is also discussed with the examination of the neck.

Excess mobility of the spine is rare. It is most easily demonstrated with the patient in the supine position. Place one hand beneath the head and the other under the knees. As the spine is flexed, it feels unusually supple, and the knees may easily approximate the chin. It occurs with those states that produce generalized hypotonia, such as Down syndrome, the amyotonias, and Ehlers-Danlos syndrome, and is sometimes seen in small children with acute potassium deficiency.

Winged scapulae occur when the lower borders of the scapulae extend out loosely from the back with excess mobility. Mild degrees occur often, but marked winging may be attributed to weakness of the muscles around the scapula. This weakness may occur after injury to the long thoracic nerve, with the muscular dystrophies, or with congenital anomalies such as absence of the clavicle (cleidocranial dysostosis) and high scapula with webbed neck (Sprengel's deformity).

Note *posture*. Lordosis and kyphosis are exaggerations of the normal anteroposterior curvatures of the spine. Lumbar lordosis is normal in children throughout childhood and appears to exist in children with protuberant abdomens. Marked lordosis may be caused by rickets, muscular dystrophy, or weakness of the abdominal wall. Adolescent round back is seen with chronic poor posture and thoracic epiphysitis.

Kyphosis is a sharp anteroposterior angulation of the spine opposite in direction to lordosis. It is usually caused by small or collapsed vertebral bodies. It is seen with tuberculosis of the spine, but it may be a diagnostic sign of mucopolysaccharidosis, Morquio's disease, or aseptic necrosis of the vertebral bodies. Localized kyphosis (gibbus) is caused by disease of one or two vertebral bodies and may occur with the same disease states causing kyphosis. Lack of normal thoracic kyphosis may thrust the heart anteriorly, known as the *straight back syndrome*.

Detect *scoliosis,* a lateral curvature of the spine. Scoliosis is detected by having the patient stand erect, marking the tips of the spinous processes with ink. Note the deviation of these ink spots from a straight line when the patient stands upright while barebacked or in a plain tight-fitting top and then bends forward with the knees straight and the arms hanging down. Structural scoliosis exists when (1) there is a double curvature with rotation (twisting) on the convexity; (2) the ink line does not straighten when the patient bends forward; or (3) one hip appears prominent. Note scapular asymmetry resulting from cervical or thoracic curves. Ask the child to bend forward. Posterior ribs should be symmetric. A lump of one group of ribs indicates structural scoliosis (Figure 7-9).

Mild scoliosis usually has no rotation, straightens in the prone position, and is related to poor postural habits. Scoliosis in a child under 5 years of age is usually attributed to congenital anomalies or to lung or chest pathologic conditions. In older children, scoliosis may be idiopathic or caused by a difference in leg length, hemivertebrae, rickets, poliomyelitis, muscular dystrophies, or neurologic disorders such as neurofibromatosis. Some curving of the lower spine is noted in children with acute abdominal pathologic conditions such as appendicitis or pyelonephritis. Painful scoliosis, which is relieved by aspirin, is suggestive of osteoid osteoma.

Figure 7-9
Forward bend is fastest way to detect scoliosis. Ribs rise. (Adapted from
Netter F: CIBA Clinical Symposia 30:1978.)

MUSCLES

Note the muscles for *development,* tenderness, *spasm,* and *paralysis.* Muscle
tone is caused by a balance between muscle mass and nerve stimulation.
It represents the degree of contraction in the voluntarily relaxed muscle.
Test muscle tone by grasping the muscle and estimating its firmness;
watch the muscle response during its normal range of motion with and
without resistance, such as response to painful stimuli in the region acti-
vated by the muscle. Note muscle strength in the older child by having the
child perform the usual function against resistance supplied by your hand.

Muscle tone is decreased in children with general debility, malnutrition, the congenital and postviral myopathic conditions, the neuropathic
conditions, carnitine deficiency, tick paralysis, some types of cerebral
palsy, lower motor neuron and cerebellar lesions, and other metabolic
diseases, including errors in glycogen and lipid metabolism. It is decreased in children with poliomyelitis, hypothyroidism, hypopituitarism,
Down syndrome, hypoadrenalism, hypokalemia, mercury and heavy
metal poisoning, and the collagen diseases. Psuedoweakness is common
in hysterical states.

Muscle tone is increased in any condition causing muscle spasm. Muscle spasm is felt as unusual tenseness of the muscle mass and may occur with injury or infection of the muscle, bone, or joint; with metabolic diseases; or with upper motor neuron lesions. Muscle spasm is also noted in diseases affecting the spinal cord roots, probably secondary to pain as in poliomyelitis. Spasm may occasionallly occur before pain, as in children with tumors of the cauda equina or in patients with abnormalities of the filum terminale, where hamstring spasm is seen early.

Generalized spasm may be seen early, involving almost all striated muscles in children with tetanus. Spasm is especially noted with slight disturbances in the environment. The generalized extensor spasm noted with tetanus can be distinguished from the generalized muscle spasm of phenothiazine intoxication. The latter does not ordinarily involve the abdominal muscles, but in tetanus the abdomen may be boardlike in its rigidity. Generalized flexion or extension spasm may be noted in children with anoxia and is seen in sickle cell crisis, presumably secondary to local muscle anoxia.

Elicit carpopedal spasm. This is elicited by restricting the blood supply to the hand or foot by (1) applying a blood pressure cuff inflated to the level of the systolic pressure or (2) applying a tourniquet or hand around the wrist or ankle for 1 or 2 minutes. Spasm of the muscles of the hands or feet with marked flexion of the wrists and ankles and extension of the fingers and toes occurs. The sign is especially prominent in children with tetany.

Note paresis, weakness, or paralysis. *Paresis* generally refers to weakness of a muscle resulting from partial paralysis, and the term *paralysis* is usually reserved for complete paralysis. These are demonstrated by the patient's inability to use a muscle after a command or painful stimulus or by observing the patient trying to use a particular group of muscles and noting a lack of motion when certain characteristic movements are attempted. Paresis and paralysis may be either spastic or flaccid.

Flaccidity, or flaccid paralysis, refers to the inability of a muscle to maintain its normal tone and position so that it yields readily and without resistance to pressure. The muscles in which it occurs should be noted. Flaccidity usually indicates lower motor neuron lesion and occurs in problems such as poliomyelitis, amyotonia congenita, myasthenia, tick paralysis, polyneuritis transverse myelitis, diabetic neuropathy, some drug and heavy metal intoxications, and spinal cord injury. Flaccidity of the lower limbs occurs with thoracic neuroblastoma resulting from extension of the tumor into the spinal canal. Paralysis that comes and goes, periodic paralysis, may be related to potassium deficiency or excess. Diastematomyelia, a spur of bone in the spinal canal, causes progressive flaccid paralysis usually during growth spurts.

The proximal muscles are usually affected first in the muscle dystrophies of adults, whereas primary neurologic disease first affects the distal muscles. This distinction is not as clear in children. Proximal muscle weakness in children is likely from muscle or anterior horn cell disease. Children who rise from the supine position by climbing up themselves instead of jumping up may have proximal muscle weakness of the pelvic muscles. Likewise, they will push themselves up to get out of chairs. Strength in the shoulder girdle can be tested by lifting children under the axillae. If the shoulder muscles are weak, children will slip through examiners' arms. Flaccidity may be caused by damage of a small area of the cerebral cortex or of the lateral hemispheres of the cerebellum; these lesions occur rarely in childhood. It is noteworthy that, as in adults with brain injury, the paralysis after the upper motor neuron lesion is first flaccid and later spastic. This is also the case in newborns with brain damage; the child may be flaccid for as long as 6 months before spasticity becomes fixed.

Paresis may also occur with chronic wasting disease, congenital heart disease, rickets, and other forms of malnutrition. Mild paresis may be noted in children with hyperthyroidism. Normally a child can hold the leg extended on command for about 1 minute; a child with hyperthyroidism can hold it about 10 seconds. Unilateral flaccidity may be noted in children with hemichorea. The leg withdraws on pinprick, distinguishing this from true paralysis. Paralysis without other neurologic signs may result from hysteria.

In infants, weakness is usually proximal in both myopathic and neuropathic conditions. In children with polyneuritis the proximal muscles are weaker in the legs, and the distal muscles are weaker in the arms. In children with pyramidal lesions, weakness in flexion is greater than that of extension in the legs, but weakness of extension is greater than that of flexion in the arms.

Spasticity refers to a prolonged and steady contraction of the muscle. It is demonstrated by increased resistance to passive movement and gives way suddenly when overcome—clasp-knife rigidity. It is accompanied by increased reflexes and clonus. Note the muscles in which it exists. Spasticity of a limb occurs with any upper motor neuron disease or after a prolonged painful stimulus. Spasticity is also marked in children with the degenerative brain diseases discussed earlier in this section. Spasticity of the extensor muscles of the legs or exaggeration of the postural reflexes with flexor spasticity in the upper extremities is more marked in children with brain damage limited to the motor cortex. However, spasticity of the extensors of both the arms and legs, or quadriplegia and tetraplegia, usually indicates more extensive damage in the cortex and the basal ganglia. Spasticity largely of the lower extremities (as in spastic diplegia) is thus usually accompanied by better mental development. Paraplegia (spasticity of the legs with no involvement of the arms) is usually caused by spinal cord disease. Diplegia is paralysis affecting the same parts on both sides of the body, usually applied to the lower limbs. Paraplegia refers to the lower limbs. Quadriplegia is paralysis of all four limbs but in usage refers to the upper limbs.

Rigidity refers to an absolute inability to flex a joint and is noted in diseases in which there is fusion of the joint. Rigidity of the neck is also noted in children with meningitis and other lesions mentioned in the discussion of the neck. Rigidity of the spine is noted in children with meningitis and other lesions discussed in the section about the spine. Usually the tendon reflexes are absent because of excessive rigidity.

Rigidity with arms flexed, legs extended, and hands fisted in the child in deep coma indicates severe dysfunction of the cerebral cortex (decorticate rigidity). Rigid extension and pronation of the arms and legs are signs of midbrain dysfunction (decerebrate rigidity).

Cogwheel rigidity of the leg muscles, manifested by spasm followed by weakness after flexion, is characteristic of children with myotonia congenita (Thomsen's disease). Good strength in the quadriceps muscles rapidly followed by weakness is noted in children with hyperthyroidism. A strong handgrip followed by weakness is seen especially in children with chorea.

Contractures are observed as fixed deformities of the muscle with limitation of joint motion, frequently accompanied by muscle atrophy. Contractures may occur in any state causing continuous spasm or disease of the muscle.

Muscle *atrophy* is best determined either by noting an obvious decrease in muscle mass or, preferably, by measuring the muscle area and comparing with the opposite side. The latter can be done on the extremities, but care must be taken that the area measured be exactly the same bilaterally. For example, if you suspect atrophy of the calf muscles of one side, measure the circumference of the calf on both sides, exactly the same distance above the malleoli.

Muscle atrophy may occur after prolonged spasm or disuse from any cause, including immobilization, malnutrition, joint disease, nervous system lesion, and the muscular dystrophies. Fasciculations of the muscles are noted as brief repetitive twitches in muscles at rest and are increased by movement of or pressure on the muscle. Fasciculations can be augmented by the administration of neostigmine, 1.0 mg, and atropine, 0.6 mg. They are usually noted in progressive lower motor neuron disease but not myopathic conditions.

Facial *myokymia* (spontaneous undulating waves of contracting muscle fibers spreading across facial muscles) appears most commonly with multiple sclerosis and intramedullary pontine tumors.

Muscle *hypertrophy* is recognized as enlarged musculature with good tone. It is usually compensatory, and other muscles are found to be atrophic. It may result from normal exercise or from constant activity, as in choreoathetosis. In pseudohypertrophy the muscle appears large because of fatty infiltration; such muscles are weak.

Muscle *percussion* is useful in distinguishing myopathic conditions from lower motor neuron disease. Briskly tap the deltoid, quadriceps, or gastrocnemius belly. Normally the muscle contracts. Response is usually normal in children with neuropathic conditions but is absent in those with myopathic conditions.

8

NEUROLOGIC EXAMINATION

AS PREVIOUSLY MENTIONED, neuropsychiatric examination is important in the examination of the child who is not acutely ill. Since the CNS is one of the most common sites of infection in the infant, this type of examination is especially important in the acutely ill infant. Remember that in addition to careful observation and neurologic examination, a detailed history of the child's development and behavior is necessary for the neurologic evaluation.

The neurologic examination of the child differs from that of the adult because the neurologic lesions usually sought in the child differ from those in the adult. For example, poisonings, congenital malformations of the brain, progressive brain diseases, and infections are common in children, whereas local vascular lesions are rare. Acute brain injury may be present in both children and adults, but bleeding in children's brains may be accompanied by delayed onset of signs because of the distensibility of the skull. In children, as in adults, metabolic diseases may also often give CNS signs. At the conclusion of the neurologic examination, you should have a good evaluation of the child's mental status and speech, cranial nerves, muscle coordination and control, and reflex sensory and autonomic functions.

Perform the neurologic examination, except for such overall procedures as the mass reflexes, with the general physical examination of each particular part of the body. Listed here are only the mass reflexes, the reflexes found in the extremities, and general aspects of the neurologic examination. However, the neurologic examination may be repeated as a whole after the general physical examination—especially if any variants are found or if neurologic difficulties are suspected—and may be recorded separately.

More important than the examination of reflexes (except in the child who is acutely ill with a neurologic disorder) is the *general impression* you get of the patient's *abilities* and *responsiveness.*

Although older children and adolescents may be examined in a manner similar to that used for adults, the infant and younger child are examined largely by observation of the characteristic *positions* of the patient, the *spontaneous movements,* and the *play activity.* Some of these qualities are discussed in Chapter 3 and in Chapter 7. You must use not only patience but also imagination in your approach to the younger patient to elicit this information. Especially in infants, compare motor and social accomplishments with suitable developmental charts (Appendix B), which with full realization of the wide variability of normals, help indicate neurologic adequacy.

Note the *state of consciousness.* The patient may be hyperirritable, convulsive, hyporeactive, delirious, stuporous, or comatose. State of consciousness may be difficult to quantitate. Responses to commands, speech, name, pinprick, or severe pain are some of the usual tests for degree of consciousness. Lack of response in the above order indicates decreasing consciousness and increasing stupor or coma. In deep coma a patient's respirations, blood pressures, and reflexes are depressed (Table 8-1). Coma with focal signs and increased reflex activity is usually caused by a brain lesion; coma with multifocal signs and decreased reflexes is usually caused by a metabolic disease or poisoning. Touch the child's eyelash lightly on either side with no warning. The child with feigned coma responds with a vigorous bilateral blink.

Generalized hyperirritability with hyperactivity in a child is usually a sign of psychologic difficulty. This response can frequently be elicited by

TABLE 8-1

Glascow coma scale*

Eye opening	Verbal	Motor	Score
		Follows commands	6
	Oriented	Localized pain	5
Spontaneous	Confused	Withdraws from pain	4
To speech	Inappropriate words	Abnormal flexion	3
To pain	Nonspecific sounds	Extension	2
None	None	None	1

*Add one number for each activity. Numbers 13 to 15 correspond to drowsiness; 10 to 12, stupor; 7 to 9, light coma; 4 to 6, deep coma; 3, flaccid and apneic. Scale is useful for following progression and regression.

SEIZURE TYPES

Partial (focal hemisphere involvement)
  Simple (consciousness not impaired)
  Complex (consciousness impaired) with or
    without secondary generalization
Generalized (bi-hemisphere involvement)
  Tonic/clonic
  Tonic
  Clonic
  Absence
  Atonic
  Myoclonic

---

observing the patient make quick movements when asked, for example, to draw a picture. Irritability may, however, be prominent in any child with an acute febrile illness, corneal abrasion, hyponatremia, hypoglycemia, chalasia with esophagitis, hernias, thrush, hair around a toe, DPT immunization, or other disease states such as acrodynia or scurvy. It may also indicate CNS disorders. Hyperactivity also occurs in children with chorea or hyperthyroidism, hypocalcemia, and other metabolic disorders. Ordinarily, younger children will be more irritable when lying on the bed or examining table than when in their mothers' arms because of a natural fear of the unfamiliar surroundings. Some infants will be more irritable when in their mothers' arms. This paradoxical irritability should alert you to the possibility of CNS infections, particularly meningitis, though other disease states such as acrodynia, scurvy, severe febrile illness, fractures, and emotional disturbances may also manifest this sign.

Convulsive states (see box) are signs of disease and should never be considered diagnoses. Seizures manifest themselves in different ways. Record the type of seizure, the parts of the body involved, and the duration.

Partial simple seizures are focal with normal consciousness and may be motor or sensory. Complex partial seizures (psychomotor, temporal lobe) may be characterized by alterations in consciousness and abnormal motor activity. Generalized seizures may be completely incoordinated tonic and clonic movements in unconscious children and may be caused by abnormal cortical discharges. Absence (petit mal) seizures are brain disturbances causing loss of consciousness for 5 to 15 seconds and are also accompanied by abnormal electrical brain discharges. Autonomic manifestations may consist of bizarre visceral disturbances and usually last longer than 30 seconds, followed by an impaired consciousness, hallucinations, total amnesia, confusion, headache, and sometimes incontinence.

Most childhood seizures begin on one side and may be thought to be focal, but they quickly become generalized, and the etiology is usually that of a generalized seizure. Cortical or subcortical irritability probably causes all types of seizures. The causes of the irritability may include many types of metabolic, vascular, or CNS disorders. Seizures do not usually occur in children with brain tumors until the intracranial pressure is considerably elevated.

Distinguish seizures from simple fainting (syncope). The latter is a sudden loss of consciousness without abnormal movements and is usually caused by reflex vascular disorders. Seizures must also be distinguished from hysterical fits, which are usually not accompanied by injuries or other neurologic signs and may contain periods during which the hysterical child is responsive. Seizures preceded by crying or cyanosis are commonly associated with breath-holding spells. Opisthotonos is more common with breath holding. Syncopal episodes occur suddenly; they may result from cardiac dysrhythmias with premonitory sensation. They occur more commonly when the child is sitting, standing, or coughing. Seizures can occur when the child is lying down or when the child has cardiac dysrhythmias, mitral valve prolapse, gastroesophageal reflux, migraine, or Tourette's syndrome. Seizures resulting from vagal-mediated cardiac arrest can be produced by 10 seconds of pressure on the eyeballs.

Lack of total activity, demonstrated by the persistence of one position for long periods, is common in mentally or emotionally delayed children or may be a sign of severe debility, malnutrition, or anemia. Catatonia, in which one unusual or apparently uncomfortable position is assumed for a long time, may be seen in mentally delayed or psychotic children. Catatonialike observation of the fingers and hands is normal in the 3- to 6-month-old child.

Lack of all activity is usually caused by a state of unconsciousness—stupor or coma—and must be differentiated from normal sleep states from which the patient can easily be aroused.

In the older child, look for other neurologic evaluations before the reflexes are elicited. Note the patient's gait, stance, limp, or ataxia, as described in Chapter 7.

Note *coordination*. Incoordination may be caused by cerebellar lesions or by any of the diseases that cause ataxia. Watch the child reach for a toy, tear paper, tie shoes, and button a shirt. Coordination is easily tested by playing a game with the child. Sit opposite the child with the child's palms upward and ask the child to strike first your right and then left hand. Continue at a rapid pace, and then shift the position of your hands. Inability of the child to follow the motion of the hands may indicate varying degrees of incoordination.

Coordination may also be tested by the finger-to-nose or heel-to-shin tests in the child who can understand commands. In these tests, tell the patient to extend first one hand and touch the tip of the nose with the index finger. This action is then repeated with the opposite hand, usually after a demonstration. The test is then repeated after the patient is told to do the same procedure with the eyes shut. Gross incoordination will be noted as the failure of the patient to touch the nose with the eyes open. Minor evidence of incoordination, as well as lack of sense of position, will be manifested by the patient's inability to perform these tests with the eyes shut. Remember that fine coordination is not fully developed in children until 4 or even 6 years of age, and if the younger patient can bring a finger within 3 or 4 cm of the tip of the nose, it is generally considered normal.

The heel-to-shin test is performed by telling the patient to run the heel of one foot down the anterior aspect of the tibia of the other foot. Usually you also demonstrate this to the patient. Inability to perform this test is a less reliable guide to evidence of incoordination or lack of position sense in a child, but tests with the eyes open and shut are similar in significance to those of the finger-to-nose test. Romberg's sign is also a test of sense of position. Fear and anxiety may result in apparent poor coordination. When asked to jump rope, some anxious children will demonstrate superior coordination and balance when jumping rope two footed or one footed and even with the eyes closed. Ask the child to hop. Inability to hop after the age of 5 indicates lack of gross motor coordination.

Note *tremors* and distinguish them from choreiform movements (Table 8-2). Tremors are constant, small movements; some occur when the patient is at rest because of lesions of the extrapyramidal system, and some occur only when voluntary motion of the part is attempted (intention tremor). Intention tremors result from lesions of the cerebellum. Tremors in the infant are seen with states of hypocalcemia and hypoglycemia. Muscular tremors or fibrillations may be noted when certain muscles are fatigued and in children with hyperthyroidism, hypothermia, hyperthermia, or progressive degeneration of the cord. Most commonly, however, tremors or twitchings may occur in infants in bursts, without obvious cause.

TABLE 8-2

Involuntary movements

Type	Character
Athetosis	Slow, continuous, writhing
Chorea	Random, jerky
Dystonia	Slow, twisting mingled with muscle tension
Fasciculation	Coarse twitching
Fibrillation	Rapid twitch in muscle fibrillation
Hemiballismus	Flinging, jumping wild, unilateral
Jack-knife	Body bends at waist (see myoclonic)
Myoclonic	Sudden, brief, shocklike
Myokymia	Twitching of muscle fibers
Spasm	Prolonged muscle contraction
Tardive dyskinesia	Writhing, fibrillation of tongue and face
Tics	Involuntary muscle contractions, noises, words
Tremor	Fine or coarse shaking
Twitch	Spasmodic, short

Twitchings (tics) are spasmodic movements of short duration, noted in muscles that are fatigued or in which a nerve is regenerating or in chorea. Twitchings may occur following sharp pain to an area. In emotionally upset children, they follow a definite and usually periodic pattern. In children with Tourette's syndrome, the twitchings increase in frequency and develop vocal bursts.

Choreiform movements are coarse, involuntary, purposeless movements associated with decreased muscle tone. They are quick, jerky, and irregular movements, grossly incoordinated, and they may disappear with relaxation. In chorea associated with rheumatic fever, choreiform movements may involve any muscle, including those of the tongue, speech, hands, and feet. These movements are best elicited by having the patient extend a hand or perform other voluntary acts. The fingers and wrists will hyperextend, and the choreiform movements of the fingers become exaggerated. With extension of the arms above the head, the palms of the hand point outward and the hand is flexed at the wrist with extension of metacarpal and interphalangeal joints. Choreiform movements are also noted in patients with hereditary ataxias and with drug reactions. Choreiform movements may be one sided (hemichorea) and, in rare cases, are caused by vascular brain lesions (hemiballismus). Paroxysmal choreoathetosis occurs after startle, lasts less than a minute, and recurs several times per week; the cause is unknown.

Athetosis refers to a group of constant, gross incoordinated movements that are slow and writhing and are usually associated with increased muscle tone. These movements are exaggerated by voluntary activity and disappear when the patient relaxes during sleep. *Dystonia* is a slow, twisting movement of limbs or trunk. Athetosis usually indicates basal ganglia involvement; ataxia and incoordination occur with even superficial cerebellar lesions. Athetoid movements may occur in children with cerebral palsy or tuberous sclerosis and is present late in the downward course of the reticuloendothelial diseases such as Niemann-Pick and Tay-Sachs. Infants may normally have athetotic movements during their first year of life.

A periodic nodding of the head (spasmus nutans) resembles athetosis. It may be idiopathic; may occur as a habit spasm; or may be a sign of mental deficiency, tumors near the optic chiasm or third ventricle, neuroblastoma, or gastroesophageal reflux. The nodding is a combination of true anteroposterior nodding and lateral shaking, which may be temporarily interrupted by suddenly attracting the child's attention. Infants with spasmus nutans usually also tilt the head and have nystagmus. To-and-fro motions of the head synchronous with the pulse (Musset's sign) may occur with aortic insufficiency.

Note *associated* movements—voluntary movements of one muscle accompanied by involuntary movements of another muscle—regulated by the cerebellum. They occur as mirror movements in the Klippel-Feil syndrome, in diseases with increased intracranial pressure, and in patients whose handedness has been changed. Reciprocal movements occur normally in infants between 2 to 4 months of age and usually decrease by 4 to 6 months of age; failure of these movements to appear or disappear at the proper times is an indication of brain damage. Certain reciprocal movements such as the movement of the arms when a person walks are normal at all ages, and their absence may indicate cerebellar damage.

Rigidity, spasticity, pareses, and paralysis are described in Chapter 7. Note handedness by observing the preferential handling of small objects. Definite handedness in a child less than 15 months old suggests hemiparesis.

The *superficial reflexes* are the abdominals, the cremasterics, and the skin reflex of the anus, which have previously been discussed. Reflexes may be reinforced by having the child grasp the examiner's hand or by moving other parts of the child's body.

Obtain the *deep tendon reflexes* of the extremities by briskly tapping the biceps, triceps, patella, and Achilles tendons with the flat of the finger. Usually a hammer or stick is used, but only with the older child.

Patients should be relaxed; you should talk casually to them or perhaps catch them unaware to best elicit these reflexes. The muscle to be stimulated should be able to act at maximal mechanical advantage; usually this is a position of about half flexion of the joint involved. Examination of these reflexes, though easy to obtain and rarely forgotten, are only a small part of the neurologic examination of the child. Tendon reflexes are stretch reflexes and are elicited by a rapid stretch of the muscle. They are elicited only in the presence of intact sensory nerves from the muscle to the spinal cord, intact nerves in the spinal cord, and intact motor nerves from the cord to the muscle. The knee jerk is usually present at birth and is followed by the Achilles and brachial reflexes. The triceps reflex should be present in children at 6 months of age.

Hyperactive deep tendon reflexes indicate upper motor neuron lesion, hyperthyroidism, hypocalcemia, or brain stem tumor and may also occur in areas of muscle spasm, such as early poliomyelitis. Hypoactive, or absent reflexes, are found in the amyotonic or myasthenic muscular dystrophies or lower motor neuron lesions, including polyneuropathy. Patients with cerebellar tumors usually have decreased reflexes. Knee reflexes may be lost early in diphtheria or later in polyneuritis. Decreased reflexes are frequently associated with flaccidity or flaccid paralysis. Flaccidity associated with active reflexes may be seen in children with some forms of brain injury, Down syndrome, malnutrition, and some disorders of amino acid metabolism. A normal contraction with delayed relaxation of the knee and ankle jerks may occur in children with hypothyroidism. Progressive extension of the leg on successive tapping of the patellar tendon (pendular knee jerk), resulting from failure of the leg to return to the resting position, occurs in chorea.

Clonus is a series of forced alternating contractions and partial relaxations of the same muscle and represents an exaggeration of hyperactive deep tendon reflexes. It may be demonstrated as a persistence of a rhythmic reflex after a stimulus (such as striking the tendon with a hammer) has been withdrawn; ordinarily, a reflex exhausts itself for a few seconds after it is once obtained. If the clonus occurs with further stimulation, it is said to be *sustained*. If repeated stimulation is necessary, it is *unsustained*. It may occur with fatigue or any of the diseases causing hyperactive reflexes.

Clonus of the knee is most easily obtained with the lower leg swinging freely over the bed or examining table while the patient is in the sitting position. Elicit the patellar reflex in the usual manner. A hyperactive knee jerk is usually obtained, and clonus exists if the patella or the muscles around the knee joint continue to contract and relax, causing the lower leg to jerk forward and back repeatedly. Clonus of the knee may also occur if the knee is flexed. Grasp the leg above the knee with one hand and the leg below the knee with your other hand; quickly push your lower hand against your upper hand. You will either feel or see the rapid contractions and relaxations.

Clonus of the ankle is best obtained by having the child lie down, with the knee flexed slightly, and the ankle resting comfortably with the toes pointing outward and upward. Hold the lower ankle lightly with your left hand, and tap the tendon with the second finger of your right hand or the hammer. Feel either the reflex or the clonic movement in the left hand. If clonus is not elicited, place the leg flat on the table with the toes pointing upward; flex the ankle quickly. Feel clonus in the hand causing the flexion.

As a group, increased muscle tone, increased tendon reflexes, clonus, spasticity, rigidity, and abnormal pyramidal tract signs are indications that point to upper motor neuron lesions, though all these signs may be seen in some metabolic disorders.

Myoclonic jerks are brief involuntary contractures of muscles. Myoclonic seizures, sometimes called *infantile spasms,* usually represent severe CNS disorders and may be an early sign of tuberous sclerosis.

In the infant under 5 months of age, *Moro's* reflex is extremely informative (Table 8-3). Elicit it by startling the patient—either by making a loud noise, dropping and catching the patient, or otherwise surprising the patient. Normally the child reacts as if grasping a tree: the arms first extend, then flex; the hands clench; and the knees and hips flex.

Absence of Moro's reflex in a newborn infant indicates severe CNS injury or deficiency. Persistent Moro's reflex after 7 months of age has the same significance. Absence of this reflex of one arm indicates frac-

TABLE 8-3
Infantile reflexes

Reflex	Appearance	Disappearance
Suck	Birth	Through infancy
Root	Birth	3-4 mo
Moro's	Birth	3-7 mo
Tonic neck	Birth	3-5 mo
Babinski's	Birth	12-24 mo
Stepping	Birth	3-4 mo
Placing	Birth	10-12 mo
Landau	3 mo	12-24 mo
Parachute	7-9 mo	Indefinite

tured humerus, brachial nerve palsy, or recently fractured clavicle. Absence of or irregular Moro's reflex of one leg indicates lower spinal injury, myelomeningocele, avulsion of the cord, or dislocated hip. Hyperactive Moro's reflex indicates tetany, tetanus, or CNS infection.

A "reverse" Moro's reflex consists of extending and externally rotating the arms, with rigidity following the usual stimulus. Such a reflex is seen in children over 5 days old who have basal ganglia disease, including kernicterus of erythroblastosis fetalis. Such children may have no Moro's reflex within the first 5 days of life.

Elicit the *Landau* reflex by supporting the infant horizontally in the prone position. The infant raises the head and arches the back. This is normally elicited from 3 months to 1½ years of age. It represents a combination of labyrinth, neck, and visual reactions; its absence suggests motor weakness, upper motor neuron disease, or mental retardation.

Obtain *Babinski's* reflex by scratching the soles of the feet with something such as a broken, pointed tongue depressor. Normally, the small toes do not move and the great toe moves plantarwise. An abnormal response is when the toes fan out and the great toe moves dorsally. The abnormal response is found in most normal children younger than 18 months of age. Persistence beyond the age of 2 to 2½ years indicates pyramidal tract lesion. Sometimes you may find it difficult to decide whether Babinski's reflex is present or absent, since only part of the response will be obtained. In such cases, look for other signs of upper motor neuron lesions before concluding that the response is abnormal. Obtain Oppenheim's sign by pressing on the median aspect of the ankle and noting the toes as in Babinski's sign. The significance is the same. Obtain Hoffmann's sign by snapping the terminal phalanx of the second finger and noting flexion of the first and third fingers. It, too, usually indicates a pyramidal tract lesion but is also obtained in children with tetany.

Kernig's sign is the inability to extend the leg with the hip flexed. This sign indicates irritation of the meninges, or hamstring spasm. Evaluation in infants under 6 months of age is difficult.

Obtain *Romberg's* sign by having the patient stand with the heels together and the eyes shut. Normally the patient is able to stand without falling. The sign is said to be *positive* if the child leans toward or falls toward one side. It occurs in children with poor or absent sense of position and in those with the cerebellar ataxias. It is also found in patients with vestibular damage and cerebellar tumors.

Foerster's symptom is obtained in children with generalized hypotonicity. Such children are sometimes called *floppy infants*. Raise the child by the armpits. The legs straighten as the child is raised if the hypotonia results from diseases with paralytic weakness such as the Werdnig-Hoffmann disease or benign variants of it; the congenital myopathic conditions—nemaline, central core, and others; metabolic disorders (for example, glycogenoses, rickets, and the muscular dystrophies); other CNS disorders; the hypotonia-obesity syndrome of Prader-Willi; connective tissue diseases; and acute illnesses. If the hypotonia results from atonic spastic diplegia, the knees and hips remain flexed.

Obtain *Trousseau's* sign by obstructing the blood flow at the wrist or ankle by making a ring around the area with the thumb and index finger or by using the blood pressure cuff. After 3 minutes, carpal or pedal spasm is produced. This sign is present in children with tetany, hyperirritability, or hyperventilation. Obtain the *peroneal* sign by tapping the lateral surface of the fibula just below the head, and note dorsiflexion and abduction of the foot. It is also seen in children with diseases of hyperirritability. These signs, in contrast to Chvostek's sign described with the examination of the face, can be obtained even in a crying child and may be helpful in diagnosing hypocalcemia.

Obtain the *grasp reflex* by placing a small object in contact with the infant's fingers. The infant will grasp the object tightly with the fingers. This movement is normally present from 1 to 3 months of age. If the movement is absent, brain or local nerve or muscle injury should be suspected. Presence after 4 months of age suggests a frontal lobe lesion. With injury to the brachial plexus, the fingers may be constantly maintained (spasticity) in the grasping position or may be flaccid. The hands are normally held as a fist for the first 3 months of life, then begin to be held open for longer periods. At approximately 6 months the normal infant should begin to take objects with one hand; at approximately 7 months of age, the infant should be able to transfer objects from one hand to the other. After 9 months of age, the infant should grasp with the fingers and appose the fingers with the thumb, and at 10 months of age the infant should develop purposeful release. These responses are delayed in children with mental dysfunction or lesions of the pyramidal tract.

The *thumb position* itself is important in determining neurologic lesions in infancy. In normal infants the thumb is in a fist in a straight line with the index finger or is freely movable in the palm of the hand. The thumb may be forcibly abducted in the palm of the hand in infants with upper motor neuron lesions.

Evaluate overall developmental motor activity. Delayed appearance of normal motor activity may be caused by brain damage, peripheral motor damage, emotional or mental delay, parental neglect or lack of challenge to the infant, prolonged illnesses, or anemia.

The 1-month-old child should be able to support the head for an instant. By 4 months of age the infant should be able to hold the head up well and roll from the supine to the prone position. At approximately 6 or 7 months of age the infant begins to sit and is able to roll over completely. At 9 months of age the infant creeps and at about 1 year of age stands with support. The infant walks at about 14 months, runs stiffly at about 18 months and runs well at about 2 years of age. Children usually cannot skip or throw a ball overhand well until about 4 years of age. For estimation of level of overall developmental motor activity, consult suitable charts or books of growth and development. The importance of the head and chest circumferences, neck and spine mobility, and the status of the fontanels as part of the neurologic examination are discussed in Chapter 4. A convenient table for following the developmental progress of infants has been systematized and should become part of each infant's record (Appendix B).

Sensory changes are difficult to determine in early childhood because of lack of cooperation. Smell and taste, using suitable stimuli, are almost never tested in the young. Blindness and deafness have previously been discussed. Of the peripheral nerves, testing is almost entirely limited to the perception of pain in the infant. Pain sensation is normal in children with muscle diseases and altered in some with neuropathies. Test for peripheral nerve injuries in the limbs by immersing the limbs in warm water for 10 minutes. The skin on the normal side wrinkles; the denervated skin remains smooth. For hand injury, check light touch sensation of the finger tips.

Withdrawal reflexes, which are obtained by applying a mildly painful stimulus and observing an unusually rapid withdrawal, usually indicate hyperesthesia and may indicate extensive lesions in the spinal cord. Hyperesthesia is noted early in children with infectious diseases of the CNS, diseases with increased intracranial pressure, peritonitis, and herpes zoster, and other diseases. Decreased sensation may be noted in children with cord or peripheral nerve lesions, mental deficiency, decreased consciousness, or such states as familial autonomic dysfunction, ectodermal dysplasia, syringomyelia, and congenital indifference to pain. When infants are held erect with the soles of the feet flat on a tabletop, they will take regular alternating steps, exhibiting the *stepping reflex*. Similarly, when prone on a tabletop with the head erect, the infant will make crawling movements. These reflex movements should disappear around 5 months of age.

In the child 6 years of age or older, obtain other sensory responses. Sense of position is described with coordination. You can test vibratory

TABLE 8-4

Some neurologic soft signs

Physical sign	Concern after age
Clumsiness in fine motor coordination	
Button 2 buttons	6 yr
Tie shoelaces	7 yr
Alternate left-right, index finger-to-nose	7 yr
Finger tapping—each finger with thumb, alternating	8 yr
Rapid alternating movements of hands (also watch for mirror movements)	10 yr
Choreiform movements, tremor	Any age
Gross motor	
Hop	6 yr
Skip	6 yr
Jump	7 yr
Toe walk	7 yr
Heel walk	7 yr
Catch ball, one hand	10 yr
Tandem gait	7 yr
Turning head with eyes	5 yr
Balance on toes	12 yr
Sensory	
Right-left orientation	5 yr
Perceive touch and identify site	6 yr
Graphesthesia, recognize numbers traced	8 yr
Recognize objects in hands	5 yr

sensations with a tuning fork. Determine astereognosis by asking the child to identify coins or other familiar objects when the eyes are shut. Test *temperature* sensation by asking the patient which end of the reflex hammer is cooler when the eyes are shut. The rubber end is usually warmer than the metal end. Cotton may be used to determine areas of decreased sensation to *touch*. Loss of any or all of these modalities of sensation may be caused by mental delay or decreased states of consciousness. In the absence of these, abnormal sensory response usually indicates posterior spinal cord root, peripheral nerve lesions, or possibly an emotional disturbance.

The other cranial nerves may be tested as a group proceeding from I to XII. The method of testing response is detailed with an examination of the head and neck in Chapter 4.

Other nonneurologic measurements, such as the character of the pulse, respiration, and blood pressure, may again be noted here as part of the central control of these functions.

Respirations are shallow and irregular with respiratory center involvement. The pulse is weak, rapid, and irregular; the skin is flushed; and the blood pressure is elevated (but may fall later) with circulatory center involvement. Not only infections and mass lesions cause involvement of the cranial centers; drugs, poisons, acidosis, alkalosis, and water balance may also affect these centers.

A group of these signs has been collated as "soft" neurologic signs, which may indicate delay in or injury to neurologic development (Table 8-4). These signs are all normal at an early age. Note the child's behavior as the child comes into the room and the child's mannerisms and behavior during the interview. Note how the child handles buttons, sleeves, buckles, and zippers. Note ease of onset of frustration and impulsivity.

Finally, note total response of the child, including cooperation, backwardness, lethargy, and reaction to physician and parent. These may be recorded in the first statement of your write-up of general appearance. Special characteristics of mental development may also be recorded here.

9

EXAMINATION OF
THE NEWBORN

The baby figure
of the giant mass
Of things to come.

William Shakespeare, *"Troilus and Cressida," Act I, Sc. 3*

THE INFANT IS a complete individual. Again, the question you want answered is, "Is the infant normal?" Even minor abnormalities should be explained to the mother to allay her fears. In the apparently well infant a second physical examination should be completed after the infant has adjusted to the new environment, since some physical abnormalities may become apparent after several days of life. However, at the first examination you are restricted to gross physical anomalies. Conduct a more thorough examination 1 to 4 hours later. You should have an exact idea of what you want to know, proceed with the examination expeditiously, and write it up if even on a checksheet. The baby should be kept warm and preferably unclothed. If the patient is not crying, listen to the chest first. Otherwise, proceed systematically from the head downward. In general, the first examination of the infant is chiefly observation of orifices and of masses, bulges, or anomalies, but the method of examination is similar to that already described in older children.

GENERAL

Note the *color* and *breathing* of the baby. If the baby is gray or cyanotic or if the respirations are labored, do not begin the examination until the airway is gently but rapidly cleared, oxygen has been given, and respiration has become regular. If in clearing the airway of mucus and amniotic fluid, a soft feeding catheter with suction is passed first through the nares into the nasopharynx and then down the esophagus to the stomach and no obstruction is met, the diagnoses of choanal atresia, esophageal atresia, and other nasopharyngeal anomalies such as nasal cysts, encephaloceles, and tumors are eliminated. Pass the catheter swiftly and gently without jerking, or laryngospasm may be induced. The tip of the catheter will be seen or felt throughout the left half of the abdominal wall. If the catheter is not palpable, cardiospasm may be present. If the catheter is down but not palpable, hold the hand over the abdomen and blow a quick puff of air through the catheter. The air bubble will be felt. If obstruction is met or the bubble is not felt, atresia in either of these areas must be considered as a possible cause of the infant's respiratory difficulty. Auscultating over the stomach while blowing air in may be deceptive, since transmitted sounds may be heard even though obstruction is present.

With the catheter in the stomach, aspirate the gastric fluid. Note the amount and quality. Normal amniotic fluid measures 5 to 25 ml and is cloudy white. Bloody fluid suggests placenta previa. Green fluid suggests meconium-stained amniotic fluid from antepartum asphyxia. More than 25 ml of fluid suggests gastrointestinal tract obstruction.

If distress persists after clearing the upper airway, maneuver a proper size laryngoscope carefully into the vallecula with the left hand, elevating the larynx by pressure with the left fifth finger on the thyroid cartilage; gently push the tongue out of the way with the blade, exposing the larynx.

Shock in an infant is usually caused by heavy sedation of the mother before delivery or intracranial trauma, but it may also result from generalized trauma of delivery, placental bleeding, a ruptured viscus, or hemorrhage in the adrenal area.

Maternal overmedication is a possible diagnosis in a depressed infant who is not meconium stained but has pallor or cyanosis, a slow, strong, full pulse, and a cord filled with blood. Asphyxia is suggested in a depressed infant who is meconium stained and pale with a slow irregular pulse; soft, distant heart sounds; and an umbilical stump that is limp and contains little blood. Lethargy after the first days is a critical sign of infection, hyperammonemia, and other metabolic disorders.

A helpful evaluation of the baby at 1 minute and at 5 minutes of life is the Apgar score, the baby's first report card. Five criteria are noted, and each is given 0, 1, or 2 points (Table 9-1). A score of 8 to 10 is excellent, 4 to 7 is guarded, and 0 to 3 is critical. Intubate the baby if the score is less than 5. Keep the baby warm.

Gross anomalies such as anencephaly, omphalocele, exstrophy of the bladder, and amelia are immediately obvious; record them in as much de-

TABLE 9-1

Apgar Score

Criterion*	Score		
	0	1	2
Color (appearance)	Blue	Fair	Pink
Heart rate (pulse)	0	100	100–140
Reflex irritability (grimace)	0	Fair	Good
Muscle tone (activity)	Flaccid	Fair or increased	Good
Breathing and cry (respiratory effort)	Apnea, 1-2 gasps	Fair	Prompt, lusty

*A score of 8 to 10 is excellent, 4 to 7 is guarded, and 0 to 3 is critical.

tail as possible. Observe the baby for symmetry of head, body, and extremities. Limbs of the term infant are flexed. Failure to move or asymmetrical movement suggests neurologic, muscle, or skeletal injury.

SKIN

Note consistency and hydration of the skin. Normally soon after birth the infant becomes pink and cries lustily. *Cyanosis* in the infant is produced by the same biochemical factors as in the older child. Because the infant usually has a higher hemoglobin level than the older child, cyanosis occurs more easily and with less relative oxygen unsaturation than in an older child (Chapter 3). Occasionally, ecchymoses will be confused with cyanosis. Pressure on a cyanotic area will blanch the skin temporarily; the ecchymotic area remains blue with pressure. Mongolian spots are usually easily distinguished from cyanosis, especially by their location.

An infant who remains cyanotic may have amniotic fluid, stomach contents, or tumors of the tongue or about the mouth obstructing the airway and causing hypoventilation. Upper airway obstruction may also be caused by choanal atresia; vascular ring; laryngeal web or cyst; or hypoplasia of the mandible with glossoptosis, tracheomalacia, vocal cord paresis, or injury to the cricothyroid cartilage.

Persistent cyanosis indicates CNS, heart, or lung disease; differentiating between these at an early age is difficult. Cyanosis in an infant with a slow cardiac or respiratory rate, with a bulging fontanel, or with limpness, especially after a rapid delivery (or of a mother who has been heavily sedated), suggests intracranial injury of the baby.

Cyanosis that lessens when the infant cries, especially if the infant is in a high-oxygen atmosphere, suggests the presence of pulmonary disease, such as respiratory distress syndrome, diaphragmatic hernia, pneumonia, asphyxia, or atelectasis. Pulmonary insufficiency is the usual cause of cyanosis in the infant. Increasing inspired oxygen is more likely to increase oxygen saturation in lung disease than in heart disease. Cyanosis that increases when the infant cries suggests cardiac disease. This test of the influence of crying on the depth of cyanosis distinguishes that resulting only from heart or lung disease. Crying should not be induced in any infant suspected of having brain injury, since the increased intracranial pressure may aggravate intracranial hemorrhage.

Localized cyanosis, which may persist for 24 to 48 hours, may sometimes be noted in a presenting part. Usually if a normal baby is slightly cyanotic at birth, cyanosis will be less in the hands than in the feet after about 4 hours of age. Equal cyanosis in the hands and feet after 4 hours of age suggests a pathologic cause of the cyanosis.

Peripheral cyanosis (acrocyanosis) is cyanosis of the hands and feet and suggests increased arteriovenous oxygen differences. It is associated with shock, sepsis, and low cardiac output. Central cyanosis involves the mucous membranes and suggests cardiopulmonary disease.

Cyanosis without dyspnea usually occurs with hypoglycemia or methemoglobinemia or if the baby is chilled. Infants at risk for hypoglycemia include those who have diabetic mothers or mothers who use illicit drugs; are small for gestational age; or have asphyxia, infection, metabolic diseases, or hypopituitarism. Cyanosis with little dyspnea may also occur with congenital heart lesions such as hypoplastic right heart, tetralogy of Fallot with severe pulmonary stenosis or atresia, pulmonary stenosis with an intact ventricular septum, and tricuspid anomalies. Cyanosis caused by congenital heart lesions with respiratory distress in the first few days of life requires emergency workup. These findings are present in infants with right-to-left shunts, such as transposition of the great arteries, total anomalous pulmonary venous return, hypoplastic left heart, and some cases of coarctation of the aorta.

Cyanosis from right-to-left shunt without organic heart disease may occur with persistent fetal circulation; persistent elevation of pulmonary vascular resistance maintains patency of the ductus and foramen ovale and may accompany hyperviscosity, atypical respiratory distress syndrome, or hypoglycemia. Cyanosis may occur a few hours after the birth of an apparently normal infant with persistent fetal circulation, tricuspid or mitral regurgitation, or other heart lesions. Cyanosis of the upper half of the body occurs with transposition of the great vessels with patent ductus;

cyanosis of the lower half of the body occurs with coarctation of the aorta proximal to a patent ductus.

In contrast to the older child, *pallor* in an infant almost always results from circulatory failure, anoxia, edema, or shock. Only rarely will a severe neonatal anemia without shock be manifested by pallor. An infant who remains pallid may have respiratory obstruction, cerebral anoxia, narcosis, cerebral hemorrhage, hypoglycemia, cretinism, or circulatory failure (for example, from adrenal hemorrhage). The pallor of anoxia is usually associated with bradycardia, and the pallor of shock with tachycardia. Postmature infants tend to have pallid skins. A beefy *red* skin may indicate poorly developed vasomotor reflexes or polycythemia or hypoglycemia in an infant born to a diabetic mother. Occasionally one half of the body may appear red and the other half pale—the *harlequin* color change of the infant. This condition is usually transient and of unknown significance. *Plethora* may also occur from twin-twin or maternal-fetal transfusion and in adrenogenital syndrome. Alternating pink and blue patches may be caused by transient vessel abnormalities or cutis marmorata.

Record evidence of *injuries* secondary to delivery or application of forceps. Scratches, petechiae, and ecchymoses are most frequently caused by injuries incident to delivery. However, *petechiae* and ecchymoses in the infant are also caused by sepsis, erythroblastosis fetalis, hemorrhagic disease of the infant, and thrombocytopenic purpura. Rarely, purpuric spots are a result of hemophilia or diseases such as toxoplasmosis, syphilis, and cytomegalic inclusion disease. These spots may occur in infants whose mothers had rubella during the first trimester or lupus erythematosus during the entire pregnancy.

Note any *tumors, hemangiomas, nevi,* and *skin tags.* Telangiectases, or capillary hemangiomas, are frequently found at the back of the neck, the base of the nose, the center of the forehead, on the eyelids (nevus flammeus), or on the mucous membranes and suggest hereditary hemorrhagic telangiectasia. Vascular nevi may appear over the face or head and may indicate Sturge-Weber disease lesions. Small angiomas may herald angiomas in the retina and brain (Von Hippel-Lindau disease). Pigmented nevi are common birthmarks and may appear any time during the first year of life. Depigmented areas that resemble a leaf and that flouresce may be an early sign of tuberous sclerosis. Note pigmented lesions of neurofibromatosis, cafe-au-lait spots, and freckles. Size, shape, color, and degree of protuberance should be recorded. Preauricular skin tags are often associated with severe congenital anomalies. *Scars,* usually around the mouth, may indicate congenital syphilis.

The skin of the infant normally feels puffy and edematous. Excess *edema* may be noted in premature infants; those born of diabetic, prediabetic, or edematous mothers; or in those with hydrops resulting from blood—especially Rh—incompatibility. It is rarely noted in children with abnormal salt retention, hypoproteinemia, heart failure, or gonadal dysgenesis.

Note any localized edema in a presenting part that resulted from trauma. Edema limited to the hands and feet may be a sign of neonatal tetany. Edema of the genitalia in both sexes is common, especially in those infants born by breech delivery. Edema of the anterior abdominal wall suggests perforation of a viscus with peritonitis, appendicitis, or obstructive uropathy. Asymmetric edema occurs with local vascular anomalies, thromboses, trauma, and Milroy's disease, a form of lymphedema.

Poor *turgor* and excessive wrinkling may indicate dehydration. Dehydration of the infant immediately after birth may indicate poor maternal nutrition, maternal toxemia, defective placenta, or sepsis of the infant. Large babies with good turgor may be born of mothers with diabetes or may occur in cretins.

The *vernix* caseosa, a cheesy white material, is found in the skin folds and the nailbeds. Yellow discoloration of the vernix occurs with intrauterine distress, postmaturity, hemolytic disease of the infant, and occasionally in infants born by breech presentation.

Desquamation occurs normally in all infants and may be generalized. Marked peeling and cracking of the skin occurs in dysmature infants. Small, hard scales may indicate congenital ichthyosis (known as *collodion* babies).

Redness of the skin with red pinpoint *macules* and *papules* developing in the first days of life are usually transitory rashes caused by irritation, toxicity, or unknown cause. Erythema toxicum may appear within the first 3 days of life and may be indistinguishable from miliaria (heat rash) or varicella. Erythema toxicum has a red base; miliaria does not. Neither involves palms or soles.

Examine *pustules* carefully. Pinpoint white spots, usually over the bridge of the nose, chin, or cheeks, are most frequently milia caused by retained sebum and are not true pustules. Small pustules that develop after waterdrop-like miliaria are a form of miliaria, either miliaria crystallina or miliaria pustulosa. Vesiculopustular lesions, which are shed leaving hyperpigmented macules, are transient neonatal pustular melanosis. Small pustules with surrounding red areas are diagnostic of impetigo neonatorum. If these pustules are associated with *bullae,* pemphigus is present. Pemphigus of the palms and soles of the infant suggest congenital syphilis. Tender, red, indurated areas with sharp borders from streptococcal infection are termed *erysipelas.* In the infant, erysipelas may be found near the umbilicus or at the site of a skin injury. Vesiculobullous lesions in the infant may also be a result of infection by viruses of herpes simplex, varicella, or variola-vaccinia if the mother is infected at the time of delivery. Vesicles may be a sign of incontinentia pigmenti.

Small discrete bullous patches involving the deeper layers of the skin, usually with large hemorrhagic areas, are called *epidermolysis bullosa.* Small reddish or purple areas of the skin that are hard and movable (fat necrosis) may be caused by trauma during or after delivery but may also indicate hypercalcemia. These areas with hard edges feel like small saucers or small, loose peas under the skin.

Redness, starting on the face and extending over the entire body and usually appearing in the second week of life—associated with desquamation of large patches of skin—is diagnostic of dermatitis exfoliativa (Ritter's disease). In this condition, large patches of epithelium can be removed by stroking the skin (Nikolsky's sign). Redness and desquamation in the skin folds represent *intertrigo,* usually caused by sweating and chafing but sometimes caused by fungal or other infections. Erythematous patches occur with neonatal lupus erythematosus.

Jaundice is sometimes difficult to determine in the infant. As in the older child, you look at the skin, the scleras, the mucous membranes, and the nail beds in natural daylight. Minimal jaundice in a plethoric infant may be more easily discerned by placing a glass slide on the infant's cheek. With slight pressure, the capillary blood and erythema will fade, but the yellowness caused by the jaundice will remain, making the jaundice more easily discernible. Jaundice is usually visible in the child or adult when the serum bilirubin reaches 2 mg/dl. It may not be visible in the infant until the level is 5 mg/dl, probably because there is less fat in the subcutaneous tissue in which bilirubin is soluble. Jaundice is usually not seen at birth because light is required to develop the pigment. The yellow-orange color is usually caused by unconjugated bilirubin; the yellow-green color, by conjugated bilirubin.

Jaundice in infants apparently progresses from the head to the feet. You can roughly estimate the level of serum bilirubin from the most caudal area of the body that is jaundiced (all levels are in mg/100 dl):

Head alone	5-8
Head and chest	6-12
To knees	8-16
Including arms and lower legs	10-18
Including hands and feet	15-20+

Jaundice appearing at birth or within 12 hours after birth is almost diagnostic of erythroblastosis fetalis. Jaundice after 24 hours is usually physiologic but may also be a result of erythroblastosis secondary to Rh or A-B-O incompatibility, sepsis, congenital syphilis, hemolytic icterus, bile duct obstruction, or viral hepatitis. Physiologic jaundice usually disappears in the full-term infant by the second week but may persist without obvious cause for as long as 4 weeks, especially in some breastfed infants. Persistent "physiologic" jaundice for longer than 4 weeks may be seen in infants with congenital heart disease, especially with heart failure or cretinism. Sepsis with jaundice is usually caused by staphylococci or *E. coli.* Sepsis without jaundice is usually from streptococci or pneumococci. Lethargy may be associated with jaundice from any cause.

Sweating is rare in the infant. It may be present in those with brain cortex irritation or anomalies or injuries of the sympathetic nervous system or in babies whose mothers were morphine addicts or drug abusers.

Congenital skin *anomalies* and deformities are common. A soft swelling, especially of the tongue or over the clavicle that contains fluid and transilluminates, is usually a lymphangioma or cystic hygroma. Midline cysts of the neck may be thyroglossal cysts. Small holes or defects anywhere in the neck and extending up to the ear may be branchial clefts or cysts.

Bluish pigmentation over the sacrum, buttocks, back, or occasionally extensor surfaces is termed *mongolian spots.* It results from pigment cells in the deep layers of the skin, usually disappears in later life when the superficial pigment masks them, and has no clinical significance.

Examine all skin folds to be certain that the skin moves over the underlying bone. Constricting bands, which are associated with deformity or atrophy beyond the contracture, may be hidden by the folds in the obese infant.

Ectodermal defects of the scalp are common. These usually appear as large, firm, sharply demarcated patches without hair. Look for small holes in the midline of the scalp or anywhere along the spinal column, which may be dermal sinuses. An infected area may be a cause of recurrent meningitis. A defect along this same area (aplasia cutis congenita) with hair over it is a marker of spinal dysraphism (for example, spina bifida, attachment to dura, or filum terminale). If neural structures protrude through the defect, the mass is termed an *encephalocele* if it is on the head and a *meningomyelocele* if it is over the spine.

Generalized *hardness* of the skin is termed *sclerema.* This condition may result from overcooling the infant and is more likely to occur in debilitated infants, particularly if they have marked alterations in their serum electrolyte levels. Patchy areas of induration of the skin (hidebound skin) is scleroderma and usually does not occur in infants.

NAILS

The nailbeds should be pink. Yellowing of the nail beds has the same significance as yellowing of the vernix. In black infants, increased amounts of melanin are normally found in the nail beds and near the genitalia. Absence or defects of the nails are usually congenital and a sign of either fetal alcohol syndrome, phenytoin treatment of the mother, or a form of ectodermal dysplasia. The nails may be short in premature infants and unusually long in postmature infants.

TONE

At birth the infant is usually limp, but after the first or second cry, the infant develops good muscle tone. Shortly after birth, infants flex themselves into "positions of comfort," the positions they occupied in utero. Note areas of flaccidity or spasticity .

Poor muscle *tone* in an infant a few minutes old should be regarded as a grave sign. In infants who remain limp longer than a few minutes, suspect anoxia, narcosis, CNS lesions—particularly edema or hemorrhage—vascular collapse, congenital left heart syndrome, hypoglycemia, Down syndrome, and avulsion or subdural hematoma of the cord. Infants with myasthenia gravis may be limp; they are born of mothers with the disease. However, many infants who have been limp for longer than several hours eventually appear to be normal. Cause of prolonged limpness in these infants is usually not adequately explained. Local loss of muscle tone may indicate a peripheral nerve lesion. Excess muscle tone may indicate CNS or metabolic muscular disease.

Seizures may be distinguished from normal tremulousness in that the convulsing child is usually quiet before the seizure and the tremulous child is usually active. Shortly after birth, seizures indicate hypoxic-ischemic encephalopathy, increased intracranial pressure from bleeding or infection, anomalies of the CNS, drug withdrawal, hypoglycemia, or hypocalcemia with tetany. Tetany is more common in infants having low birth weight, diabetic mothers, or asphyxia. Rarely, omphalitis resulting from *Clostridium tetani* causes tetanus of the infant with convulsions. Another rare condition, neonatal nephritis, also causes convulsions.

Muscular *twitching* and hypertonicity are similar in diagnostic significance as convulsions. However, *tremors* and twitchings of short duration may be noted, especially if the infant is cold or startled; these are usually normal and occur in active infants. Tremors of no pathologic significance cease if you place a finger in the infant's mouth and let the infant suck. Overalertness with twitching may result from narcotic withdrawal if the mother is addicted or may rarely indicate hyperthyroidism. Asymmetric seizures do not help distinguish metabolic from intracranial causes. Seizures resulting from hypocalcemia or infection usually begin after the fourth day of life; those caused by anoxia, birth injury, anomalies, or hypoglycemia begin in the first 3 days of life.

A few *facies* are characteristic at this age. Down syndrome facies can usually be recognized at birth, but cretinism is usually not detectable until about 6 weeks of age. Mucopolysaccharidoses can be detected only if suspected, since characteristic facies appear after several months. The facies of an infant with renal agenesis is characterized by low-set ears, senile appearance, broad nose, and receding chin. Major facial anomalies may indicate chromosomal abnormalities. Note multiple fractures in children with osteogenesis imperfecta. Disproportion of one side of the body indicates absence or abnormalities of the bones or muscles or congenital hypertrophy. Other facies are described in Chapter 3.

HEAD

Note carefully the presence and amount of overriding of the *sutures*. Immediately after birth the fontanels may appear to be very small or entirely closed, and the suture lines will be represented by hard ridges. These findings are normal and are considered part of the molding process of a normal vaginal delivery. Within the first day of life, normal intracranial pressure begins to exert its expansive force, and the suture lines and fontanels are felt as depressions in the normal infant. The progress of this expansion is followed during the entire period of infancy but especially during the neonatal period. Failure of normal expansion in the neonatal period may be the earliest sign of microcephaly or craniostenosis. In contrast, rapid enlargement of the fontanels is not a good early sign of developing hydrocephalus; absolute measurements of skull and chest circumference are necessary for this diagnosis. Anencephaly and congenital hydrocephaly are obvious at birth. To detect hydrancephaly, hydrocephalus, or subdural hematoma, *transilluminate* the head of any infant whose head is asymmetric or unusually large or small or who has abnormal neurologic signs.

A tense *fontanel* any time after birth and until the fontanel closes indicates increased intracranial pressure. Except in those infants whose intracranial pressure is raised because of crying or coughing, a tense or bulging fontanel is usually a pediatric emergency, suggesting intracranial infection or bleeding. Estimate intracranial pressure by raising the infant's head until the fontanel is flat; then measure the vertical distance from the fontanel to the clavicle. Normally, this does not exceed 55 mm in the first few months of life.

A depressed fontanel may be normal or may be an early indication of dehydration. A third fontanel, located between the anterior and posterior fontanels, is a sign of an infant at risk.

Cephalohematoma is frequently not present at birth but appears on the second day of life. The hematoma is soft and fluctuant, and the outline is well defined with the edge at the bone margin. If the cephalohematoma crosses the midline, fracture of the skull is present. A cephalohematoma begins to calcify in the first few days of life, and a ridge around the hematoma may be felt for as long as 6 months.

In contrast to the cephalohematoma, the *caput* succedaneum is soft but ill defined in outline, pits on pressure, and is not fluctuant. The characteristics represent edema of the scalp, perhaps from pressure on the emissary veins. Record the presence of caput, since this may indicate difficult delivery with possible intracranial hemorrhage.

Press the scalp behind and above the ears with the fingers, as if playing the piano, to determine the presence of a ping-pong ball sensation, *craniotabes.* Many normal infants have craniotabes, but if it is present, hydrocephalus and syphilis should also be suspected. The other causes of craniotabes occur later in life (see Chapter 4).

Cranial or facial *asymmetry* is common and is usually caused by intrauterine molding or molding during delivery. Facial or cranial asymmetry may occur in infants with facial palsy, but usually infants with facial nerve injury are not born with asymmetry. Try to assess facial asymmetry as the infant begins to cry. Segments of the facial nerve may be injured and cause confusion; for example, the mentalis nerve and its muscle prevent drawing down the corner of the mouth but spare the nasolabial fold and palpebral fissure. This type of weakness may be permanent. Facial palsy may be hereditary. Central palsy occurs with Möbius' syndrome. Facial asymmetry may occur in infants of low birth weight and associated hemihypertrophy (Silver syndrome) and with congenital heart disease in cardiofacial syndrome. If present, *micrognathia* (small mandible) may be a cause of cyanosis. Head retraction may be a sign of a vascular ring causing respiratory obstruction. Chvostek's sign is usually positive in the normal infant and therefore of little value in diagnosing neonatal tetany.

EYES

If the infant is crying or keeps the eyes shut, gently rock the head. Usually the infant will open the eyes long enough for a thorough examination.

Note the presence, structure, and equality of the eyes. Edema of the lids may be caused by birth trauma. Real tears may not appear until the infant reaches the second month of life, and the lacrimal ducts may not open until several weeks later. Purulent discharge from the eyes that is present shortly after birth usually signifies ophthalmia neonatorum as a result of gonorrhea or *Chlamydia* infection. Although any discharge from the eyes may begin on the infant's first day of life, chemical irritation usually causes discharge on days 1 to 3, gonorrhea between days 2 to 5, and inclusion blennorrhea from viral or *Chlamydia* infection on days 4 to 14.

A mongoloid slant (the lateral upward slope of the eyes with an inner epicanthal fold) or an antimongoloid slant may be variants or may suggest one of the syndromes of mental, physical, or chromosomal aberrations. The inner canthal length is normally 1.5 to 2.5 cm, the outer canthal length is 5.0 to 7.5 cm, and the interpupillary distance is 3.0 to 4.5 cm.

Exophthalmos at this age is usually a congenital anomaly with enlargement of all the structures of the eye (buphthalmos). However, congenital glaucoma is a cause of exophthalmos in the infant. An open-eyed stare, common in infants with cerebral palsy, may be confused with exophthalmos.

Enophthalmos is usually associated with ptosis and constricted pupil (Horner's syndrome) and indicates damage to the brain or to the cervical spine and brachial plexus root at this age. Constricted *pupil* alone, unilateral dilated fixed pupil, and *nystagmus* or *strabismus* may each be an early sign of brain injury. A searching nystagmus is not uncommon at birth. Later, this type of nystagmus may indicate blindness. An intermittent strabismus is present in nearly all infants at birth but disappears by 6 months of age.

Conjunctival or scleral *hemorrhages* are common and usually have no clinical significance. They may, however, indicate difficult delivery or hemorrhagic disease of the infant. Blood in the anterior chamber (hyphema) is visible as a fluid level when the head is erect and usually indicates more extensive trauma. Conjunctival edema and discharge may appear a few days after birth and are usually caused by chemicals or eye infections.

Examine the *cornea* for anomalies of the cornea and pupil. Keratitis at this age may be due to trauma but usually signifies gonorrhea. The corneal reflex should be present at birth but is tested only if brain or eye damage is suspected. Haziness may indicate cataract or glaucoma. Congenital cataracts may indicate maternal rubella, galactosemia, or disorders of calcium metabolism.

Examine the *retina* and test for a red reflex. Raising the infant's head with one hand is often helpful in getting the infant to open the eyes long enough to visualize the retina. If you examine properly, absence of the red reflex may indicate the presence of lens opacities or retinoblastoma. Retinal hemorrhages usually indicate subdural hematoma or other brain trauma. Choreoretinitis, whitish spots on the retina resulting from congenital toxoplasmosis or cytomegalic inclusion disease, may be found.

The pupil of the infant may be constricted for about 3 weeks or may respond to light at birth by contracting, *(pupillary reflex)*. Absence of the reflex after 3 weeks suggests that the infant is blind or may have suffered intracranial anoxia or oculomotor nerve damage. The infant's eyes should follow a light. The pupil is normally black to direct light. White pupils indicate opacity in the lens, vitreous, or retina. Detect sixth nerve paralysis by watching the eye fail to move laterally as you rotate the head in the opposite direction (doll's eye maneuver).

EARS

Note anomalies, position, clefts, tags, and injuries of the external ear. Low-set ears may be associated with renal agenesis or chromosomal abnormalities. The canals are usually filled at birth with vernix and amniotic debris, so you may not visualize the drums; however, they are usually easily visualized at a few days of age. You can estimate deafness at a few days of age by snapping your fingers or making a sharp noise. Normally the eyelids will twitch or a complete Moro's reflex will be obtained. In the infant with deafness, there is no such response; suspect congenital deafness, filled aural canals, congenital syphilis, and kernicterus.

NOSE

The nose is usually deformed for a few days after birth, but injury is rare. Test patency of the nasal canals by holding your hand over the baby's mouth and noting the normal passage of air. Mucus is usually present. A more certain method of testing nasal patency is to pass a soft rubber catheter with suction, as already described. Nonpatent nasal airway at this age is usually caused by choanal atresia or other congenital anomaly. Occasionally, a tumor or encephalocele may be protruding. Nasal discharge may be present normally, and sneezing is common. Thick bloody nasal discharge without sneezing suggests congenital syphilis (snuffles). Sneezing may occur in cretins and in infants whose mothers were receiving reserpine or narcotics.

MOUTH

Note *harelip* and *cleft palate*. Always open the mouth to search for anomalies. Because of the normally high arched palate, it may be difficult to visualize the mouth beyond the uvula. Ordinarily, visualization beyond this point is not necessary. Insert a gloved finger to feel for a cleft or submucous cleft, tumors, or thyroid cyst at the base of the tongue. A large tongue usually results from tumor (lymphangioma or hemangioma). The tongue is rarely enlarged at birth in the cretin; it is large in infants with Wiedemann-Beckwith syndrome or Pompe's disease (glycogen storage disease, type II) and appears large in the Pierre Robin syndrome with micrognathia.

A protruding adderlike *tongue* is seen with brain injury. The frenulum of the tongue may be prominent but usually does not restrict motion of the tongue. Obtain the *sucking* reflex by placing the tongue blade on the lips, and stimulate the *rooting* reflex by touching the cheek and noting the infant turn and suck; both are normal reflexes present at birth. Absence of these reflexes occurs in brain-injured or debilitated infants and in some normal infants for the first day or two of life.

Teeth may be present at birth. Retention *cysts,* or pearls, are common along the gum margins. Flat white spots that do not rub away (thrush) may be present by 3 or 4 days of life. Small hard *tumors* may be seen in the gingiva, especially in the incisor area (epulis). You may see ulcers, or plaques, on the hard palate after a few days of age (Bednar's aphthae) that are usually due to vigorous sucking. Small, white epithelial cysts along both sides of the median raphe of the hard palate are Epstein's pearls. *Tonsillar* tissue is not seen in the newborn.

Vomiting is a symptom in older children but may be considered a sign in the infant. It is common in the infant of 1 or 2 days of age and may be a result of relaxation of the cardia of the stomach. It has various causes, such as cerebral anoxia, increased intracranial pressure, sepsis, marked jaundice, adrenal hyperplasia, peritonitis, intestinal obstruction from volvulus, tracheoesophageal fistula, malrotation, annular pancreas, diaphragmatic hernia, atresia of the intestine, meconium ileus, bands, diverticuli, duplications, imperforate anus, Hirschsprung's disease, cretinism, and metabolic diseases.

Vomiting of uncurdled milk or prompt vomiting of anything occurs in infants with esophageal atresia but also occurs in normal infants who have been fed too much or too fast or who have not been properly burped or positioned after feeding. Passage of a catheter with suction, as previously described, helps to determine presence of esophageal atresia. Bloody vomitus in the infant most commonly results from ingested blood, but it occasionally occurs with hemorrhagic disease of the infant or with gastrointestinal ulcers associated with intracranial anoxia or increased pressure. Vomitus with bile suggests an obstruction below the ampulla of Vater or perforation of a viscus; without bile, it suggests obstruction above the ampulla. Fecal vomiting usually indicates a low intestinal obstruction. Vomiting also occurs in children with electrolyte disturbances, urinary tract disease, and infections.

Saliva is usually scant until the second or third month of life. Profuse salivation with mucoid secretions in the infant may indicate the presence of tracheoesophageal fistula or cystic fibrosis, but it may frequently be caused by tracheal aspiration or irritation.

NECK

The infant's neck is generally not visible with the infant in the supine position. Bring the neck into full vision by placing one hand behind the upper back and allowing the head to fall gently into extension.

Distended neck veins usually signify a mass in the chest or pneumomediastinum. A mass in the lower part of the sternocleidomastoid muscle with limitation of motion of the neck results in torticollis. Small cystic masses in the region of the upper part of the sternocleidomastoid may be branchial cleft cysts. A fractured clavicle may present as a mass in the neck. A midline mass may be a congenital goiter, which is rare, or a thyroglossal duct cyst, which is more common. A soft mass over the clavicle that transilluminates may be a cystic hygroma.

An unusually short, poorly mobile neck may be an indication of the Klippel-Feil syndrome; skin folds from the acromion to the mastoid may indicate gonadal dysgenesis. Excess posterior cervical skin may indicate other chromosomal aberrations.

Flex the neck. Resistance is rare but may indicate meningeal irritation. However, lack of resistance does not indicate lack of meningeal irritation, since an infant with meningitis may have a supple neck.

Retraction (opisthotonos) may be caused by intracranial injury or infection.

Turn the neck from side to side to obtain the tonic neck reflex, which is normally present in the infant. Absence may indicate CNS damage. When the head is turned with the infant in the supine position, the trunk should rotate in the direction of the head movement (the neck-righting reflex). Similarly, if the body is tilted in the erect infant, the head should return to the upright position, a labyrinth response (otolith-righting reflex).

CRY

Note the cry of the infant. The infant should cry lustily at birth. A weak or groaning cry or grunt in expiration usually indicates severe respiratory disturbances. Absence or weakness of cry or constant crying at birth usually indicates brain injury, laryngeal anomaly, or vocal cord paresis. A high-pitched (or cerebral) cry may indicate increased intracranial pressure. Hoarseness or crowing inspirations may indicate laryngeal disease or anomalies such as laryngeal or thyroglossal tumor, mucous plugs, congenital laryngeal stridor, laryngeal paralysis, stenosis of the larynx or trachea, congenital heart disease, vascular ring, tracheomalacia, tracheal webs or other causes extrinsic to the larynx (such as diaphragmatic hernia, Pierre Robin syndrome, cystic hygroma, pneumothorax, abnormal thoracic cage, bronchogenic cyst, and mediastinal masses). Hoarseness appearing at 2 to 5 days of age frequently results from laryngospasm caused by hypocalcemia. Hoarseness is usually absent at birth in congenital laryngeal stridor; at birth, presence of hoarseness requires study.

CHEST

Examine the chest for gross anomalies, tumors, and fractures. The chest is usually almost circular. Depressed sternum may be caused by atelectasis, respiratory distress syndrome, and funnel chest. The xiphisternum protrudes and normally appears broken as a result of the xiphoid's weak attachment with the body of the sternum. Retractions usually indicate interference with air entry. Marked retraction of the chest suggests upper airway, particularly laryngeal, obstruction such as laryngeal stenosis. Immediate direct laryngoscopy is indicated.

Asymmetry of the chest may result from diaphragmatic hernia or paralysis, pneumothorax, emphysema, tension cysts, pleural effusions, pneumonia, and pulmonary agenesis. An asymmetric mass near the neck may be a fractured clavicle. Palpation may reveal congenital absence of a clavicle or of muscle (Poland's syndrome).

With a warm hand, palpate for the cardiac impulse. In a normal baby, it is barely palpable. An impulse felt in the subcostal angle or left parasternal area occurs with ventricular enlargement. Increased activity at the apex indicates left ventricular overactivity. Thrills may be felt over the aortic area or suprasternal notch with aortic stenosis, at the second left interspace with pulmonic stenosis, at the second or third left interspace near the sternum with patent ductus, and at the fourth interspace near the sternum with ventricular septal defect.

Enlargement of the *breasts* in either sex caused by maternal hormones is usually seen on the second or third day and may persist normally as long as a month. Milky secretions may normally be present. Redness and firmness around the nipple is rare and results from infection—mastitis or abscess. Increased pigmentation of the areola is found in adrenogenital syndrome. Supernumerary nipples are noted, since they may be associated with internal organ anomalies.

LUNGS

The infant's *respiration* is chiefly abdominal. Decreased abdominal respiration is noted in infants with pulmonary disease, ruptured viscus, peritonitis, or distended abdomen. Thoracic breathing or unequal motion of the chest is noted in those with phrenic nerve paralysis, diaphragmatic hernia, or massive atelectasis. Unequal motion of the chest or deep retraction of the sternum, especially if associated with rapid, gasping, or grunting respiration or flaring nares, indicates intrathoracic disease.

Respiratory *rate* is 30 to 60 breaths per minute (bpm) at birth. Respiratory movements are irregular in rate and depth in the normal infant. Periods of apnea less than 10 seconds in length may be normal. Weak, irregular, slow, or very rapid rates suggest brain damage. Rates above 60 bpm suggest pulmonary disease (as described under cyanosis) and transient tachypnea of the infant; below 30 bpm indicates apnea or intracranial injury. Tachypnea without severe dyspnea suggests phrenic nerve paralysis or methemoglobinemia.

Grunting rapid respirations may be the only sign of a very sick infant and may be caused by overwhelming infections anywhere in the body—lung, heart, or brain diseases; anemia; and distended abdomen.

Deep-sighing respirations are noted frequently in infants with acidosis. Increased depth of respiration with cyanotic heart disease results from decreased pulmonary blood flow. Deep respirations also occur with pulmonary hypertension. Decreased depth occurs with heart failure, shock, CNS diseases, and sepsis. Cheyne-Stokes respiration or weak, groaning respiration may be a sign of hypoxia or brain damage in the full-term infant. The *cough reflex* is usually absent in the infant but appears in a day or two.

During percussion or auscultation of the chest, the child must lie so that the head and neck are not turned. Increased or decreased areas of dullness or changes in breath sounds may occur simply because of the infant's position.

The chest is resonant shortly after birth. Hyperresonance suggests emphysema but is more often a result of pneumomediastinum, pneumothorax, or diaphragmatic hernia. Decreased resonance indicates improper aeration, usually caused by atelectasis and occasionally by pneumonia, respiratory distress syndrome, or empyema. Atelectasis may represent primary failure of expansion of the lung or may be a result of aspiration of amniotic fluid, food, or other foreign body; thyroid or possibly thymic tumors; other mediastinal masses; diaphragmatic hernia; or chylothorax. Pleural effusion may also be caused by chylothorax or lung disease, including pneumonia.

Auscultation should reveal bronchial breath sounds bilaterally. Air entry should be good, particularly in the midaxillary line. An expiratory grunt suggests difficult air exchange. Rales and rhonchi may be normal for the first 1 to 4 hours of life due to neonatal atelectasis. Pleuropericardial rubs have no clinical significance. Peristaltic sounds may be heard in the chest with diaphragmatic hernia, though these sounds are frequently transmitted from the abdomen in normal infants. If breath sounds are heard on both sides of the chest and the heart sounds are heard in the usual place, diaphragmatic hernia or pneumothorax is unlikely. Intrinsic lung diseases may cause changes in breath sounds.

A Downes score to estimate degree of respiratory distress in infants with no pneumothorax. pneumomediastinum, or aspiration can be obtained (Table 9-2). Such a score is useful in indicating oxygen requirements of the baby. A score of 0 to 3 represents mild distress, 4 to 6 represents moderate distress, and 7 to 10 represents severe distress.

Transilluminate with a bright cool light above and below the nipple on each side. Increased transillumination around the sternum indicates pneumomediastinum; illumination elsewhere indicates pneumothorax.

TABLE 9-2
Downes Score

Criterion	Score		
	0	1	2
Respiratory rate	<60	61-80	>80 or apneic
Cyanosis	0	In air	In 40% O_2
Retractions	0	Mild	Moderate to severe
Grunt	0	With stethoscope	Without stethoscope
Air entry (crying, axilla)	Clear	Delayed	Barely audible

HEART

Percuss to obtain heart *size* or palpate the apical impulse. The apex will usually be found lateral to the midclavicular line and in the third or fourth interspace because of the more horizontal position of the infant's heart. Beware of dextrocardia. A large heart at birth is rarely found with valvular heart disease, but it is seen in children born of diabetic mothers and those with erythroblastosis fetalis, Pompe's disease, or rhabdomyoma of the heart. A few days after birth, however, cardiac enlargement may be caused by heart failure secondary to heart anomalies (for example, coarctation of the aorta, septal defects, patent ductus arteriosus, hypoplasia of the left heart, truncus arteriosus, transposition, tricuspid or pulmonary atresia, aortic stenosis, anomalous venous return, and anomalous coronary arteries) or endocardial fibroelastosis, paroxysmal tachycardia, hypertension of any cause, or toxic myocarditis. Enlarged heart with other signs of heart failure may also be a result of peripheral arteriovenous connections, such as cerebral arteriovenous aneurysms. Pulmonary arteriovenous fistulas do not usually cause heart enlargement because of low pressure on the heart. Normal-size hearts may also occur with hypoplastic right heart, pulmonary atresia or stenosis, and tricuspid anomalies.

The heart rate at birth varies from 100 to 180 bpm and stabilizes shortly after birth at 120 to 140 bpm. The *rhythm* is usually regular. Varying rhythm is associated with anoxia, cerebral defects, increased intracranial pressure, and heart block.

Sinus arrhythmia is present in all term and most preterm infants. Absence of arrhythmia is found in infants with respiratory distress syndrome. Tachycardia of over 170 bpm after 1 hour may be because of infection, dehydration, anemia, congestive heart failure, or hyperthyroidism. Bradycardia may be a result of anoxia, CNS disease, or heart block, as in neonatal lupus syndrome.

Listen with either the bell or the diaphragm. The first and second *sounds* are almost equal. Splitting of the first sound may be caused by an ejection click from aortic or pulmonic stenosis. Wide splitting of the second sound occurs with atrial septal defect and total anomalous venous return.

Murmurs are noted for loudness, quality, location, and timing, but their significance varies at this age. Murmurs, if present, are usually heard at the left sternal border in the third or fourth interspace or over the base of the heart—almost never at the apex. For the first hour up to 15 hours of life, a late systolic or continuous murmur in the pulmonary area is presumably originating from a physiologically patent ductus arteriosus. Another innocent murmur is a short, early systolic ejection murmur with or without an early systolic click at the lower left sternal border or pulmonary area, which is loudest at 3 months of age. A third innocent murmur is a short systolic ejection murmur in the axilla and over the back. A soft systolic murmur associated with an ejection click in the pulmonary area may be caused by pulmonary disease. Loud murmurs on the first day of life suggest semilunar valve stenosis or atrioventricular valve incompetence. Loud systolic murmurs appearing between the third and seventh days of life suggest ventricular septal defect.

Heart sounds are poorly heard with pneumothorax or pneumomediastinum, cardiac failure, or CNS injury. A single second heart sound may indicate pulmonary atresia or hypoplastic left heart. Clicking or crackling sounds synchronous with the heartbeat suggest mediastinal emphysema.

ABDOMEN

The abdomen is usually prominent. The veins over the abdomen are prominent normally but are distended in infants with peritonitis and pylephlebitis.

Visible peristaltic waves indicate intestinal obstruction but may be seen in thin, otherwise normal infants. Peristalsis is normally heard shortly after birth. A silent tympanitic distended tender abdomen suggests peritonitis or necrotizing enterocolitis.

Scaphoid abdomen in infants suggests diaphragmatic hernia or high atresia of the intestinal tract. The abdomen may be distended with ascites, tumors, genitourinary obstruction, low intestinal obstruction such as atresia of the ileum or colon, imperforate anus or meconium plug, peritonitis or ileus, sepsis, meconium ileus, tracheoesophageal fistula, omphalocele, gastroschisis, enlargement of abdominal organs, pneumoperitoneum, and Hirschsprung's disease.

Ascites may result from any of the causes listed under edema, ruptured viscus, chylous ascites, peritonitis, necrotizing enterocolitis, hepatitis, cirrhosis, congenital anomalies causing obstruction of the portal vein or urethra, or other genitourinary anomalies.

The *liver* is normally palpated 2 to 3 cm below the right costal margin. The *spleen* tip is usually palpable around 1 week of age. Enlarged liver and spleen are usually palpated or percussed in infants with erythroblastosis fetalis, heart failure, sepsis, trauma to liver or spleen, neuroblastoma, or congenital syphilis. Enlarged liver and spleen are also found in infants born of diabetic mothers and sometimes in those with congenital hemolytic icterus. A liver extending far below the costal margin in the midline, yet not palpable laterally, may result from partial herniation of the left lobe of the liver into the infant's chest with left-sided diaphragmatic hernia.

Left-sided liver is usually associated with situs inversus. Other malrotations are usually not detected by physical examination. The lower half of the right and the tip of the left *kidney* are normally palpated. You cannot diagnose agenesis of the kidney, however, just because the kidney is not felt. If the infant is crying, palpation for the kidneys may be facilitated by supporting the infant at a 45-degree angle with one hand at the occiput and neck. Palpate the abdomen with the free hand, and simultaneously flex the neck with the other hand. Abdominal muscles will relax, and the infant usually stops crying. Flexing the knees to the abdomen sometimes also gives enough relaxation. Both kidneys are palpable and are about 3 to 5 cm in length.

Most flank *masses* are of renal origin. Enlarged kidneys may be noted with neuroblastoma, Wilms' tumor, polycystic kidneys, or congenital hydronephrosis. A single, enlarged kidney may indicate renal vein thrombosis. The abnormal kidney mass most frequently palpated in the abdomen results from multicystic renal dysplasia, a common form of cystic disease of the neonatal kidney.

The *bladder* is normally percussed or palpated 1 to 4 cm above the symphysis. Ironically, a greatly distended bladder in the infant is palpated with difficulty because of its very thin wall; it must be percussed or it will be overlooked. Distended bladder may result from congenital bladder-neck or urethral obstruction.

Any other masses palpable in the abdomen must be identified. Tumors, meconium ileus, loculated hemorrhage, or other abnormal masses may be found.

Inspect the umbilical *cord*. If the amnion covers the umbilical stump, the condition is called *amniotic navel;* if covered by skin, it is *cutis navel*. Neither has any clinical significance except that the former may be associated with delayed healing and the latter may be mistaken for umbilical hernia. A velamentous cord with insertion near the edge is rare but may signify other anomalies. The umbilical cord normally has two arteries; examine for this because a single artery may be accompanied by other anomalies, particularly renal abnormalities or chromosomal trisomies. The artery is thick walled; the vein is thin walled.

The cord should be dry and not bleeding. If it is bleeding, the cord must be retied. Redness around the cord after 24 hours, wetness of the stump, or a fetid odor after 3 days usually signifies the presence of omphalitis. A cord that fails to drop off after 2 weeks or a navel that persists in draining after 3 weeks may indicate the presence of a urachal cyst or sinus. Similarly, a child born with a very large and flabby umbilical cord may have a patent urachus. Fecal discharge occurs with a persistent omphalomesenteric duct; this usually indicates Meckel's diverticulum. Patent omphalomesenteric duct may result in ileal prolapse, a surgical emergency.

Soft granulation tissue is commonly seen following cord separation. This local condition must be distinguished from the firmer umbilical polyp, which is dark red, has a mucoid discharge, and is related to Meckel's diverticulum. Other cysts and tumors of the umbilicus occur rarely.

Ventral *hernias,* with or without diastasis recti, are frequently present at birth and are usually insignificant. Very large hernias (omphalocele) may be incompatible with life. Occasionally a child is born with a hernia that pinches off the small bowel. Omphaloceles are midline, covered by a sac. Gastroschisis is a paramedian defect, usually on the right with no sac. An umbilicus that shifts with respiration (belly-dancer's sign) signals phrenic nerve paralysis.

GENITALIA

Inspect the genitalia. Edema is common, especially in infants born by breech delivery. Pigmentation is usually increased around the genitalia in dark-skinned races (for example, Blacks, people of Mediterranean descent, and Hispanics) but may be a sign of adrenal hyperplasia. Note *femoral pulses, hydrocele,* and hernia. Though the clitoris is always large, carefully inspect the labia. An unusually large clitoris and partial or total labial fusion are found in pseudohermaphroditism, usually caused by adrenal hyperplasia. What appears to be a large clitoris may be a small penis. Micropenis (a penis less than 2 cm in length) may be a sign of other organ anomalies. Identify the urethral opening. In the female infant the urethral opening is just back of the clitoris. In the male infant, if the opening is on the ventral surface of the penis, hypospadias exists; if it is on the dorsal surface, epispadias is present. Ulceration of the urethral orifice may occur in the infant, especially following circumcision.

A tight *prepuce* is usually found in infant males; phimosis does not exist unless the prepuce cannot be pulled back just far enough to allow the flow of a good urinary stream. Do not retract the prepuce more than is adequate for examination. Small bands and adhesions of the prepuce usually break during the examination. Erection and even priapism may be noted in the infant but are usually without clinical significance.

Palpate the *testes*, whether they are in the canal or scrotum. The scrotum may appear large or bruised, especially after breech delivery. Dark hematoma in the scrotum may indicate rupture of the liver. A deep cleft in the scrotum results in a bifid scrotum, frequently associated with other genitourinary anomalies. Note hydroceles and hernias. A unilateral, dark, swollen, nontender testis may be a sign of testicular infarction of the infant.

The vulva is hyperemic. The *labia*, especially the labia minora, are usually large in the infant female. The normal labia may be confused with a bifid scrotum. Palpate the labia majora for a small body, which may be a gonad. Adhesions of the labia minora may occur shortly after birth. Because of maternal hormones, vaginal mucoid or bloody *discharge* may occur normally in the female any time in the first week and may persist as long as a month. A catheter can again be used. Visualize the opening of the hymen. Passing the catheter through the hymenal opening tests for imperforate hymen and vaginal atresia. Polyps or caruncles of the hymen may be present. These regress spontaneously. The normal uterus may be felt; it is about 2 cm in length. Palpate for femoral pulses; absence suggests coarctation of the aorta. Fecal urethral discharges may be present. They indicate rectourethral, rectovaginal, or rectovesical fistulas.

SPINE

Now place the infant in the prone position. Run your hand lightly over the spine. Spina bifida, pilonidal sinus, scoliosis, and the anal dimple are sought. If the *anus* does not appear patent, insert the previously used catheter. If the abdomen is distended, perform the rectal examination immediately. Anorectal anomalies, including displacement of the anus, may be associated with saccrococcygeal teratoma. Prominence of one buttock with asymmetric gluteal folds and an abdominal mass indicates an internal saccrococcygeal teratoma.

MECONIUM AND URINE

Although it usually is not considered part of the physical examination, the passage of meconium and urine should be noted. The infant usually voids immediately at or within a short time of birth. Failure to pass urine by 24 hours of age is highly suggestive of urinary tract obstruction or other urinary tract anomaly and requires further investigation.

Meconium is usually passed during the first 3 days of life. Passage of meconium before birth is diagnostic of fetal intrauterine distress. Failure of passage of meconium by the end of the second day of life suggests an intestinal tract obstruction, including stenosis or atresia anywhere through the length of the intestinal tract, meconium ileus, megacolon, or small left colon syndrome in infants of diabetic mothers.

Passage of small amounts of meconium or passage over a long time suggests a high intestinal or partial intestinal obstruction. Presence of bright red blood in the meconium is usually from the baby ingesting mother's blood, but it may be from hemorrhage somewhere in the intestinal tract, for example, necrotizing enterocolitis with or without perforation—an emergency distinction that suitable laboratory tests must determine.

EXTREMITIES

Place the infant in the supine position. Gently fold the infant into the infant's intrauterine position, encouraging relaxation and maybe even sleep. This position also provides a clue to the range of motion normal to that child. For example, a child whose hips and knees are drawn to one side in utero will have a greater range of motion of the abducted hip than the adducted hip. Count the fingers. Note polydactyly and syndactyly. Feel for fractures, paralyses, and dislocations of the clavicles and upper extremities. Examine the hips for dislocation by rotating the thighs with the knees flexed. Soft clicks are common when hips are moved, as described in Chapter 7. These must be distinguished from the sharp click of dislocation. Clicks at the knees are also common.

Multiple fractures with deformity may be a result of osteogenesis imperfecta. Paralysis of the arm may be from brachial palsy or fractured humerus. Paralysis of both legs is usually caused by severe trauma or congenital anomaly of the spinal cord. The hands are normally held clenched. The thumb is in the hand like a fist but moves out intermittently. Permanent fisting signifies a cortical thumb resulting from cortical spinal tract injury.

Test the *grasp* reflex. On pulling upright, the head is normally partially supported. Elbows, hips, and knees generally lack full extension. Response to pain and touch are noted but ordinarily not recorded. Note the tone of the muscle groups. Test passive tonus by moving all the major joints. Paralysis, missed during examination of tone, may be detected. Look for septic arthritis or osteomyelitis in any septic neonate. Examine other nerve and muscle injuries as described for the older child.

Palpate the radial *pulses*. Increased right compared with left radial pulse occurs with supravalvular aortic stenosis or juxtaductal coarctation. Alternate strong and weak pulses (pulsus alternans) is a sign of left ventricular failure. Paradoxical pulse (pulsus paradoxicus), in which the pulse changes markedly with respiration, occurs with cardiac tamponade or constrictive pericarditis.

Edema of the extremities may be caused by heart failure and liver diseases and other causes of hydrops such as blood incompatibility, chorioangioma of the placenta, umbilical or chorionic vein thrombosis, fetal neuroblastoma, cystic adenomatoid malformation of the lung, pulmonary lymphangiectasia, Chaga's disease, fetal Gaucher's disease, and local vascular abnormalities.

MEASUREMENTS

Measure and record the head, chest, and abdominal circumferences and the length of the infant. At birth the head should be at least 0.5 cm larger than the chest or abdomen. If there is any question about developing hydrocephalus, repeat measurements at daily intervals.

Take the temperature by rectum with the infant in the prone position or in the axilla, groin, or other areas if indicated. Temperatures of 33° C to 34° C (92° F to 94° F) are common in the infant and rise when the infant is warmed. Low temperatures are also noted after severe birth trauma and severe infection. Aural temperatures are higher than rectal or esophageal temperatures due to brain metabolism. Lower aural temperatures suggest hydranencephaly.

Elevated temperatures are noted frequently in the infant who is dehydrated, when brain damage or sepsis occurs, and when the environmental temperature is excessively high. If the temperature elevation at the feet and abdomen is almost the same, the fever is usually caused by the environment; if the temperature of the feet is low and that of the abdomen high, sepsis is more likely.

NEUROLOGIC STATUS

Finally, the infant's crib is slapped or dropped a few inches and Moro's reflex (Chapter 8) is carefully observed. This response, or the lack of it, is valuable in determining CNS status, fractures of the arms and legs, brachial plexus injury, congenital dislocation of the hip, and recent fracture of the clavicle. An infant with fractured clavicle may move the arm freely after 24 hours. In infants with Erb's palsy the arm hangs limply, with internal rotation at the shoulder and pronation of the lower segment, and does not move as a result of paralysis after brachial plexus injury. In pseudo Erb's palsy, decrease in passive as well as active motion indicates an injury to the proximal humeral epiphysis. Moro's reflex is absent at birth and improves in infants with cerebral edema. Moro's reflex may be present at birth and disappear in infants with cerebral hemorrhage.

Alternatively, Perez's sign, another mass reflex, may be obtained. With the baby prone on a hard surface, exert thumb pressure over the spine from the pelvis to the neck. A strong cry will be noted in the normal infant, together with flexion of the lower and upper extremities, lordosis of the spine, elevation of the pelvis and head, and urination and defecation. Its significance is similar to that of Moro's reflex.

Before leaving the delivery room, inspect and weigh the *placenta.* Amnion nodosum or vernix granuloma may reflect insufficiency of amniotic fluid as in Potter's syndrome.

Polyhydramnios (excess amniotic fluid) occurs in infants of diabetic, preeclamptic, or anemic mothers; in multiple pregnancies; and in infants with anencephaly, gastrointestinal obstruction, erythroblastosis, tracheoesophageal fistula, and anomalies of the great vessels. *Oligohydramnios* occurs with agenesis of or polycystic kidneys.

EXAMINATION OF THE LOW-BIRTH-WEIGHT NEWBORN

A baby is God's opinion
that the world should go on.

Carl Sandburg

A low-birth-weight (LBW) infant is one who weighs less than 5.5 lb (2500 g) at birth. Infants with LBW may be premature (less than 37 weeks gestational age), with size appropriate for gestational age (AGA), small for gestational age (SGA), or postmature with weight loss from placental insufficiency.

When an LBW infant is examined, the same principles are followed as for the examination of the full-term infant. The examination must be even more rapid and less complete and, above all, performed gently and tenderly in a warm protected area.

Measurements of the head, chest, abdomen, length, and weight; observation for gross abnormalities; and rapid estimation of air exchange, heart rate, and skin texture usually suffice for the initial examination. Accurate measurements assist in properly estimating gestational age. If a temperature measurement is desired, it should be taken in the axilla; temperatures of premature infants approximate that of the environment. Examination to determine the presence of Moro's reflex may be deferred until the infant is more than a day old and then performed only by rapping the crib side. Transillumination of the head, if performed, will show large areas of light transmission.

Calculate the *ponderal index:*

$$\frac{wt\ (g)\ \times\ 100}{length\ (cm)^3}$$

Less than 2.3 g/cm^3 is small; 2.3 to 2.7 g/cm^3 is normal. A small ponderal index is associated with increased neonatal and sometimes persistent complications.

Normal respiration in a premature infant is irregular and Cheyne-Stokes in type. The average rate varies from 40 to 80 bpm. A slow rate, rarely a rapid rate, or a regular respiratory rate usually indicates CNS depression. A rapid rate is more frequently a prime indication of respiratory distress syndrome; infection (usually generalized), including omphalitis, meningitis, septicemia, and pneumonia; or atelectasis.

Because the bony thorax is soft, each inspiration is marked by indrawing the sternum. This collapse of the sternum normally lessens in the first 24 hours and disappears no later than the fourth or fifth day of life. Persistence of the indrawing suggests the presence of persistent atelectasis. Marked atelectasis is usually present at birth but diminishes with each breath. Frequently, an infant does well for a few minutes or a few hours and then shows signs of respiratory distress, including marked collapse of the chest wall, rapid respiratory rates, grunting, and cyanosis. Respiratory distress syndrome, foreign material aspiration with secondary atelectasis, pneumothorax, infection (especially with group B streptococci), severe primary atelectasis, pneumomediastinum, and localized emphysema or reopening of the ductus arteriosus with subsequent pulmonary edema should be suspected. Apparently severe respiratory distress with tachypnea, which clears in 1 to 2 days, is benign transient tachypnea of the infant. The cough reflex is usually absent in the premature infant.

Cyanosis in a premature infant usually disappears within a few minutes of birth. Persistent cyanosis is similar in significance to that in a full-term infant.

Note the texture of the skin. The skin of the premature infant is thin and extremely tender; it is subject to easy bruising, bleeding, and infection and is more subject to injury by temperature changes (which result in hardening [sclerema]) than the skin of the full-term infant.

Certain physical signs are characteristic of normal premature AGA infants: a typically round head larger than the chest, prominent eyes, absence of eyebrows and lashes, absence of sweat, purple mottling of the skin (cutis marmorata), extensive hair (lanugo) over much of the body, and soft nails. The neck and extremities are short; the head, hands, and feet are prominent; labia minora are prominent; and the abdomen appears full. Peristalsis is normally visible through the thin abdominal wall, and it is usually not an indication of obstruction. Bloody vomitus in a premature infant may be caused by intracranial hemorrhage, peptic ulcer, necrotizing enterocolitis, or swallowed blood.

Although premature infants may remain edematous for 4 or 5 days, they usually remain dehydrated longer than the full-term infant. As soon as the edema fluid is absorbed, the skin of the premature baby becomes and remains wrinkled. Jaundice appears and disappears slowly. Many premature infants have umbilical hernias, and the incidence of other hernias, especially inguinal, is higher in premature than in full-term infants. A large number of premature infants have capillary hemangiomas.

The normal premature infant may seem almost motionless for the first 3 or 4 days after birth. Decreased tone, especially in the SGA infant, suggests hypoglycemia. Then the child begins to cry and make vigorous movements for a few minutes at a time. Early movements usually correspond to the time of disappearance of edema and probably to the onset of hunger. The cry is usually high pitched in the normal premature child.

The degree of prematurity can sometimes be estimated by measurements of length, weight, and head circumference (Figure 9-1) and their comparison with those of a term infant. Attempt to estimate gestational

Text continued on p. 208.

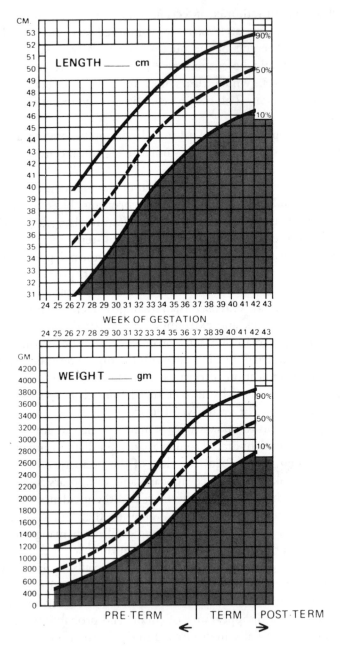

Figure 9-1
Classification of newborns, based on maturity and intrauterine growth.
*(From Lubchenco LC, Hansman C, and Boyd E: J Pediatr 37:403, 1966;
Battaglia FC and Lubchenco LC: J Pediatr 71:159, 1967.)*

	1st Exam (X)	2nd Exam (O)
LARGE FOR GESTATIONAL AGE **(LGA)**		
APPROPRIATE FOR GESTATIONAL AGE **(AGA)**		
SMALL FOR GESTATIONAL AGE **(SGA)**		
Age at Exam	hrs	hrs
Signature of Examiner	M.D.	M.D.

Figure 9-1, cont'd

NEUROMUSCULAR MATURITY

	0	1	2	3	4	5
Posture						
Square Window (Wrist)	90°	60°	45°	30°	0°	
Arm Recoil	180°		100°·180°	90°·100°	< 90°	
Popliteal Angle	180°	160°	130°	110°	90°	< 90°
Scarf Sign						
Heel to Ear						

PHYSICAL MATURITY

	0	1	2	3	4	5
SKIN	gelatinous red, transparent	smooth pink, visible veins	superficial peeling &/or rash, few veins	cracking pale area, rare veins	parchment, deep cracking, no vessels	leathery, cracked, wrinkled
LANUGO	none	abundant	thinning	bald areas	mostly bald	
PLANTAR CREASES	no crease	faint red marks	anterior transverse crease only	creases ant. 2/3	creases cover entire sole	
BREAST	barely percept.	flat areola, no bud	stippled areola, 1–2 mm bud	raised areola, 3–4 mm bud	full areola, 5–10 mm bud	
EAR	pinna flat, stays folded	sl. curved pinna, soft with slow recoil	well-curv. pinna, soft but ready recoil	formed & firm with instant recoil	thick cartilage, ear stiff	
GENITALS Male	scrotum empty, no rugae		testes descending, few rugae	testes down, good rugae	testes pendulous, deep rugae	
GENITALS Female	prominent clitoris & labia minora		majora & minora equally prominent	majora large, minora small	clitoris & minora completely covered	

Figure 9-2
Newborn maturity rating and classification. *(Scoring system from Ballard JL et al: A simplified assessment of gestational age,* Pediatr Res 11:374, 1977. *Figures adapted from Sweet AY: Classification of the low-birth-weight infant. In Klaus MH and Fanaroff AA, eds:* Care of the high-risk infant, *Philadelphia, 1977, WB Saunders.)*

Gestation by Dates _____ wks

Birth Date _____ Hour _____ am / pm

APGAR _____ 1 min _____ 5 min

MATURITY RATING

Score	Wks
5	26
10	28
15	30
20	32
25	34
30	36
35	38
40	40
45	42
50	44

SCORING SECTION

	1st Exam=X	2nd Exam=O
Estimating Gest Age by Maturity Rating	_____Weeks	_____Weeks
Time of Exam	Date _____ am / Hour _____pm	Date _____ am / Hour _____pm
Age at Exam	_____ Hours	_____ Hours
Signature of Examiner	_____ M.D.	_____ M.D.

Figure 9-2, cont'd

age as accurately as possible. Infants of LBW may be of decreased gestational age, or the LBW may be caused by various maternal, placental, or fetal factors. The prognoses of these two groups differ. A scoring system has been helpful in more precise determination of gestational age (Figure 9-2).

Because the incidence of severe congenital anomalies is higher in premature than in full-term infants, these anomalies must also be sought.

APPENDIX A

RECORD OF PHYSICAL EXAMINATION

Temp _____ Pulse _____ Resp _____ BP _____
Age _____ Sex _____ Ht _____ Wt _____
Head circ _____ Chest circ _____
Skin folds _____

General appearance. Ill or well, distressed, alert, cooperative, body build. Reaction to parents. Facies. Characteristic position, movements, nutrition, development. Speech.

Skin. Color, pigmentation, cyanosis. Veins, arteries, thrombophlebitis. Jaundice, carotenemia. Pallor. Eruptions. Petechiae. Ecchymosis. Hives. Dermatographia. Tache cerebrale. Subcutaneous nodules. Xanthomas. Texture. Scaling, striae, scars, sweat, subcutaneous tissue, emphysema. Turgor, edema.

Nails. Cyanosis, pallor, pulsations, pitting, hemorrhages.

Hair (body). Distribution, color.

Lymph nodes. Occipital, postauricular, cervical, parotid, submaxillary, sublingual, axillary, epitrochlear, inguinal. Size, mobility, tenderness, heat.

Head. Position, hair, shape, sutures, fontanels. Circumference. Microcephaly, hydrocephaly. Craniotabes, Macewen's sign. Percussion, sinuses. Auscultation, bruit, veins.

Face. Shape. Facial paralysis, trigeminal paralysis. Swelling; parotid, submaxillary, sublingual glands. Facial appearance, hypertelorism, twitching, Chvostek's sign.

Eyes. Vision, visual fields. Blinking. Scleras, exophthalmos, enophthalmos. Strabismus. Ocular movement. Nystagmus. Ptosis, eyelids.

Conjunctivae, pingueculae, pterygium, styes, chalazion, blepharitis. Cornea, discharge. Pupils, accommodation, iris. Retina, red reflex, fundus, vessels, hemorrhage, chorioretinitis, disc, macula. Corneal reflex.

Ears. Anomaly, position. Discharge. Tenderness. Canals. Drums, redness, light reflex, landmarks, bulging, perforation, mobility. Mastoids, nodes. Hearing. Vestibular function.

Nose. Shape. Alae nasi, flaring. Mucosa, secretions, bleeding, airway. Septum. Polyps, tumor, encephalocele. Sinuses.

Throat. Circumoral pallor.

Lips. Paralysis, cleft, fissures, vesicles, color, edema.

Mouth. Odors, trismus. Teeth, number, edges, occlusion, caries, formation, color. Salivation.

Gums. Infection, discoloration, bleeding, cysts. Buccal mucosa, thrush, veins.

Tongue. Coating, moisture, tremor, papillae, color, geographic, furrows, scars, size, tongue-tie, cysts, paralysis.

Palate. Color, bleeding, cleft, perforation, arch. Epiglottis. Uvula, soft palate. Posterior pharynx. Tonsils, infections, size. Postnasal drip. Koplik's spots, eruptions, ulcers.

Larynx. Voice. Laryngoscopy. Speech.

Neck. Size, anomalies, webbing, edema, nodes, masses. Sternocleidomastoids. Trachea. Thyroid. Vessels. Motion, opisthotonos, Brudzinski's sign, tonic neck reflex. Head drop. Tilting. Nodding.

Chest. Inspection, shape, circumference, rosary, Harrison's groove, flaring, angle, expansion; abdominal, thoracic, intercostal motion, retraction, symmetry, scapulae.

Breasts. Observation, development, symmetry, redness, heat, tenderness, masses. Tanner stage.

Lungs. Respiration. Type, Cheyne-Stokes. Rate, tachypnea, slow, apnea, Biot. Depth, hyperpnea. Dyspnea, exercise tolerance. Cough, hemoptysis, sputum, cough reflex. Palpation, masses, tenderness, thud, fremitus; interspaces, retraction, paralysis; pulsations, friction rubs, nodes. Percussion, dullness, scapulae, diaphragm, liver, heart, mediastinum, hyperresonance. Auscultation, sounds, rales, rub, slap, rhonchi, wheezes, vocal resonance, peristalsis.

Heart. Inspection, bulging, impulse; distress, cyanosis, edema, clubbing, pulsations, vessels, femoral pulse, blood pressure. Pulse rate, tachycardia, pulsus alternans, bradycardia, water-hammer, thready, dicrotic, pulsus paradoxus. Arrhythmia, premature beats, extrasystoles, rhythm, fibrillation. Palpation, size, apex impulse, tenderness, thrill. Percussion. Auscultation, sounds, quality, split, third sound, gallop, tic-tac, friction rub, venous hum, murmurs. Failure.

Abdomen. Inspection, shape, distention, transillumination, respiration. Umbilicus, diastasis, veins. Peristalsis. Gastric waves. Auscultation. Percussion, fluid, masses. Palpation, superficial, tense, tenderness, rebound; spleen, liver, masses. Deep palpation, ballottement, bladder, kidneys, reflexes. Femoral pulses, hydration, consistency.

Genitalia. Discharge, foreign body, caruncle, prolapse. Labia, adhesions, vagina, clitoris. Penis, hypospadias, epispadias, phimosis. Scrotum, testes, hydrocele, hernia. Cremasteric reflex, nodes. Tanner stage.

Anus and rectum. Buttocks. Fistula. Fissure. Prolapse. Polyps. Hemorrhoids. Diaper rash. Rectum, fistula, megacolon, masses, prostate, uterus, tenderness. Sensation.

Extremities. Anomalies, length, clubbing, pain, tenderness, temperature, gangrene, swelling, deformities, shape. Feet. Gait, stance, balance, limp, ataxia.

Spine. Hair, dimples, masses, spina bifida, tenderness, mobility. Opisthotonos, scapulae. Posture, lordosis, kyphosis, scoliosis.

Joints. Heat, tenderness, swelling, effusion, redness, motion. Hips.

Muscles. Development, tone, tenderness, spasm, paralysis, rigidity, contractures, atrophy.

Nervous system. General impression, abilities, responsiveness, position, spontaneous movements, play activity, development. State of consciousness, irritability, convulsive states. Gait, stance, limp, ataxia. Coordination. Tremors, twitching, choreiform movement, athetosis, associated movements. Rigidity, paresis, paralysis, spasticity, flaccidity. Reflexes, superficial, tendon, clonus. Moro's, tonic neck. Babinski's, Oppenheim, Hoffmann, Kernig, Romberg, Foerster, Trousseau, peroneal, Chvostek, grasp. Thumb position. Neck and spine mobility, fontanels. Sensation, blind, deaf, withdrawal reflex, hyperesthesia, hypesthesia, position, vibration, temperature, touch. Astereognosis. Cranial nerves, I to XII. Respiratory center, circulatory center.

APPENDIX B

THE DENVER II REVISION AND RESTANDARDIZATION OF THE DENVER DEVELOPMENTAL SCREENING TEST

Because services for handicapped children have markedly expanded since the Denver Developmental Screening Test (DDST) first appeared in 1967, the test has undergone a major revision and restandardization. A pool of 350 potential items was developed through a review of existing items and the creation of additional ones. Criteria for the administration and interpretation of each item were developed. The items were standardized on two samples: (1) Denver County ($N = 1039$) subdivided into three ethnic groups, each of which was further divided on the basis of maternal education. Each of these was again divided into 10 age categories; (2) the Colorado non-Denver sample ($N = 1057$) was subdivided into three residence categories (rural, suburban, urban), and each was further subdivided on the basis of maternal education and age of children similar to the Denver County sample.

Each item was examined via regression analysis to determine the age at which 25%, 50%, 75%, and 90% of children in each subgroup could perform the item. A goodness of fit test was applied to the data to determine the accuracy of the curves. Tester-observer and test-retest reliability was determined for each item.

The final selection of 125 items was made on the basis of eight criteria. Changes in times were an 86% increase in language items, the addition of two items on speech intelligibility, and a 22% decrease in the number of report items.

The 125 items are displayed on a test form that has an age scale corresponding to the AAP recommended health maintenance visits. The test form also includes a behavior rating scale (Figures B-1 and B-2).

Currently the Denver II screening manual, test form, and proficiency test are being used in diverse parts of the United States. For interpretation purposes, the *Denver II Technical Manual* contains norms of subgroups

Reprinted with the permission of Frankenburg WK and Dodds JB, University of Colorado Medical Center, Denver.

having significantly different ages at which 90% of children pass the item compared with the group norms that are presented on the test form.

Detailed administration and scoring instructions are given in the *Denver II Screening Manual,* which must be used to ensure accuracy in administration of the test. These materials are available form DDM, Inc, PO Box 6919, Denver, Col 80206-0919.

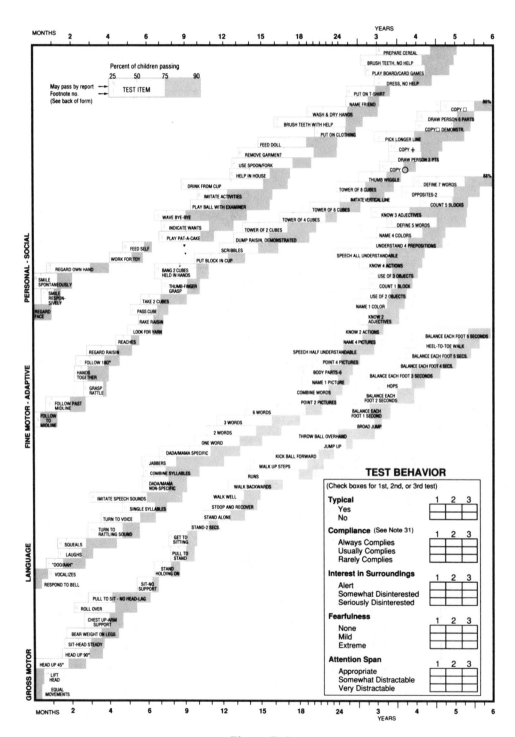

Figure B-1

DIRECTIONS FOR ADMINISTRATION

1. Try to get child to smile by smiling, talking or waving. Do not touch him/her.
2. Child must stare at hand several seconds.
3. Parent may help guide toothbrush and put toothpaste on brush.
4. Child does not have to be able to tie shoes or button/zip in the back.
5. Move yarn slowly in an arc from one side to the other, about 8" above child's face.
6. Pass if child grasps rattle when it is touched to the backs or tips of fingers.
7. Pass if child tries to see where yarn went. Yarn should be dropped quickly from sight from tester's hand without arm movement.
8. Child must transfer cube from hand to hand without help of body, mouth, or table.
9. Pass if child picks up raisin with any part of thumb and finger.
10. Line can vary only 30 degrees or less from tester's line.
11. Make a fist with thumb pointing upward and wiggle only the thumb. Pass if child imitates and does not move any fingers other than the thumb.

12. Pass any enclosed form. Fail continuous round motions.

13. Which line is longer? (Not bigger.) Turn paper upside down and repeat. (pass 3 of 3 or 5 of 6)

14. Pass any lines crossing near midpoint.

15. Have child copy first. If failed, demonstrate.

When giving items 12, 14, and 15, do not name the forms. Do not demonstrate 12 and 14.

16. When scoring, each pair (2 arms, 2 legs, etc.) counts as one part.
17. Place one cube in cup and shake gently near child's ear, but out of sight. Repeat for other ear.

18. Point to picture and have child name it. (No credit is given for sounds only.)
    If less than 4 pictures are named correctly, have child point to picture as each is named by tester.

19. Using doll, tell child: Show me the nose, eyes, ears, mouth, hands, feet, tummy, hair. Pass 6 of 8.
20. Using pictures, ask child: Which one flies?... says meow?... talks?... barks?... gallops? Pass 2 of 5, 4 of 5.
21. Ask child: What do you do when you are cold?... tired?... hungry? Pass 2 of 3, 3 of 3.
22. Ask child: What do you do with a cup? What is a chair used for? What is a pencil used for?
    Action words must be included in answers.
23. Pass if child correctly places and says how many blocks are on paper. (1, 5).
24. Tell child: Put block **on** table; **under** table; **in front of** me, **behind** me. Pass 4 of 4.
    (Do not help child by pointing, moving head or eyes.)
25. Ask child: What is a ball?... lake?... desk?... house?... banana?... curtain?... fence?... ceiling? Pass if defined in terms
    of use, shape, what it is made of, or general category (such as banana is fruit, not just yellow). Pass 5 of 8, 7 of 8.
26. Ask child: If a horse is big, a mouse is ___? If fire is hot, ice is ___? If the sun shines during the day, the moon shines
    during the ___? Pass 2 of 3.
27. Child may use wall or rail only, not person. May not crawl.
28. Child must throw ball overhand 3 feet to within arm's reach of tester.
29. Child must perform standing broad jump over width of test sheet (8 1/2 inches).
30. Tell child to walk forward, heel within 1 inch of toe. Tester may demonstrate.
    Child must walk 4 consecutive steps.
31. In the second year, half of normal children are non-compliant.

OBSERVATIONS:

Figure B-2

APPENDIX C

PHYSICAL GROWTH AND THE EARLY LANGUAGE MILESTONE SCALE

The charts of head circumference in boys and girls from the ages of 1 month to 18 years are shown in Figure C-1. Figures C-2 through C-7 show physical growth percentiles for boys and girls from birth to 18 years of age. Figures C-8 through C-10 present the early language milestone scale..

Figure C-1
Head circumference in boys and girls from 1 month to 18 years of age.

Figure C-2

Girls: Birth to 36 months physical growth NCHS percentiles.
(Modified from Hamill PVV and others: Physical growth: National Center for Health Statistics percentiles, Am J Clin Nutr 32:607-629, 1979. Data from the Fels Research Institute, Wright State University School of Medicine, Yellow Springs, Ohio. Courtesy Ross Laboratories, Columbus, Ohio.)

Figure C-3

Boys: Birth to 36 months physical growth NCHS percentiles.
(Modified from Hamill PVV and others: Physical growth: National Center for Health Statistics percentiles, Am J Clin Nutr 32:607-629, 1979. Data from the Fels Research Institute, Wright State University School of Medicine, Yellow Springs, Ohio. Courtesy Ross Laboratories, Columbus, Ohio.)

Figure C-4
Girls: 2 to 18 years physical growth NCHS percentiles. *(Modified from Hamill PVV and others: Physical growth: National Center for Health Statistics percentiles, Am J Clin Nutr 32:607-629, 1979. Data from the National Center for Health Statistics [NCHS], Hyattsville, Md.)*

Figure C-5

Girls: Prepubescent physical growth NCHS percentiles. *(Modified from Hamill PVV and others: Physical growth: National Center for Health Statistics percentiles, Am J Clin Nutr 32:607-629, 1979. Data from the National Center for Health Statistics [NCHS], Hyattsville, Md.)*

Figure C-6

Boys: 2 to 18 years physical growth NCHS percentiles. *(Modified from Hamill PVV and others: Physical growth: National Center for Health Statistics percentiles, Am J Clin Nutr 32:607-629, 1979. Data from the National Center for Health Statistics [NCHS], Hyattsville, Md.)*

Figure C-7
Boys: Prepubescent physical growth NCHS percentiles. *(Modified from Hamill PVV and others: Physical growth: National Center for Health Statistics percentiles, Am J Clin Nutr 32:607-629, 1979. Data from the National Center for Health Statistics [NCHS], Hyattsville, Md.)*

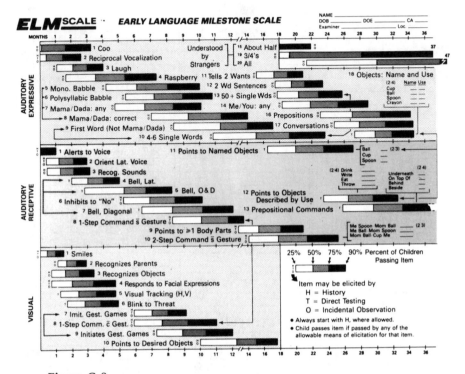

Figure C-8
The early language milestone scale. The horizontal axis is the age in months.

Figure C-9
The Early Language Milestone Scale (ELM Scale) is a tool for assessing language development from birth to 36 months of age and intelligibility of speech from birth to 48 months of age. Language is assessed independently in three areas: auditory expressive, auditory receptive, and visual. Auditory expressive development is subdivided into content (such as cooing, babbling, single words, two-word phrases) and intelligibility (clarity of speech). Auditory receptive development includes prelinguistic auditory behaviors (orienting to voice or bell), plus comprehension of progressively more complex verbal commands. Visual language includes prelinguistic behaviors (visual tracking and response to facial expressions) and symbolic features such as pointing to desired objects. Item V10 (index finger pointing) emerges at the same age as item AE 9 (first word) and implies the same degree of linguistic competence. The ELM Scale may be scored on a pass/fail basis or may be converted to point scores and percentile values for auditory expressive, auditory receptive, visual, and global language function.
(From Coplan J: The early language milestone scale, Austin, Tx, 1987, PRO-ED.)

I. General Instructions

a) Draw vertical line down entire page at child's chronologic age (CA).

b) Work *backward* from CA, until three consecutive items in each Division (AE, AR, V) are passed (=Basal Level).

c) If child achieves Basal without failing any items already attained by more than 90% of children, *stop*. ELM screen is passed.

d) If one or more items that have already been attained by more than 90% of children are failed, work *forward* from CA until three consecutive items in that Division are failed. (Exception: Child is permitted to fail *one* of the following without penalty: V3-V6). The 50% value of the highest item passed in each Division is the Ceiling Level.

If Ceiling Level ≥CA→ELM screen is passed.

If Ceiling Level <CA→ELM screen is failed.

II. Auditory Expressive (AE)

a. Content

AE1: Prolonged musical vowel sounds in a singsong fashion (ooo, aaa, etc.), *not* just grunts or squeaks.

AE2 H: "Does baby watch speaker's face and appear to listen intently, then vocalize when the speaker is quiet? Can you 'have a conversation' with your baby?"

AE4 H: Blow bubbles or "bronx cheer"?

AE5 H: Isolated sounds such as ba, da, ga, goo, etc.

AE6 H: Repetitive string of sounds: "babababa" or "lalalalala," etc.

AE7 H: Says "mama" or "dada," but uses them at other times besides just labeling parents.

AE8 H: Child *spontaneously, consistently,* and *correctly* uses "mama" or "dada," *just* to label the *appropriate* parent.

AE9, AE10 H: Child *spontaneously, consistently,* and *correctly* uses words. Do not count "mama,"

Figure C-9, cont'd

"dada," or the names of other family members or pets. *Do* list the particular words.

AE11 H: Uses single words to tell you demands. "Milk!" "Cookie!" "More!" etc. Pass = two or more wants. List specific words.

AE12 H: *Spontaneous, novel* two-word combinations ("Want cookie," "No bed," "See daddy," etc.) *Not* rotely learned phrases that have been specifically taught to the child or combinations that are really single thoughts (e.g. "hot dog").

AE14 H: Child uses "me" or "you" but may reverse them ("you want cookie" instead of "me want cookie," etc.)

AE17 H: "Can child put two or three sentences together to hold brief conversations?"

AE18 T: Put out cup, ball, crayon, and spoon. Pick up cup and say, "What is this? What do we do with it (What is it for)?" Child must *name* the object and give its use. Pass = "drink with," etc., *not* "milk" or "juice." Ball: Pass = "throw," "play with," etc. Spoon: Pass = "Eat" or "Eat with," etc., *not* "Food," "Lunch." Crayon: Pass = "Write (with)," "Color (with)," etc. Pass item if child gives *name and use* for two objects.

b. Intelligibility

AE15, AE19, AE20: "How clear are the words your child makes? That is, how much of your child's speech can a stranger understand?"
— Less than half
— About half (AE15)   Pick One
— Three quarters (AE19)   (H,O)
— All or almost all (AE20)

To Score:

If "less than half": Fail all three items in cluster

If "about half": Pass AE15 only

If "three quarters": Pass AE19 and AE15

If "all or almost all": Pass all three items in cluster

Figure C-9, cont'd

III. Auditory Receptive (AR)

AR1 H,T: Any behavioral change in response to noise (eye blink, startle, change in movements or respiration, etc.).

AR2 H,T: What does baby do when mother starts talking while out of baby's line of sight? Pass if any shift of head or eyes to voice.

AR3 H: Does baby seem to respond in a specific way to certain sounds (becomes excited at hearing parents' voices, etc.)?

AR4 T: Sit facing baby, with baby in mother's lap. Extend both arms so that your hands are behind baby's field of vision and at the level of baby's waist. Ring a 2-inch diameter bell, first with one hand, then the other. Repeat × 2 or × 3 if necessary. Pass if baby turns head to the side at least once.

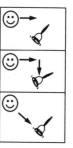

AR5 T: See note for AR4. Pass if baby turns head first to the side, then down to localize bell at least once. (Automatically passes AR4.)

AR6 H: Does baby understand the command "No" (even though baby may not always obey)?

AR6 T: Test by commanding, "*(Baby's name)*, no!" while baby is playing with any test object. Pass if baby temporarily inhibits actions.

AR7 T: See note for AR4. Pass if baby turns directly down on diagonal to localize bell at least once. (Automatically passes AR5 and AR4.)

AR8 H: Will your baby follow any verbal commands *without* you indicating by gestures what the action is ("Stop," "Come hear," "Give me," etc.)?

AR8 T: Wait until baby is playing with any test object, then say, "*(Baby's name)*, give it to me." Pass if baby extends object to you, even if baby seems to change mind and takes the object back. May repeat command × 1 or × 2. If failed, repeat the command, but this time hold out your hand for the object. If baby responds, then pass item V8 (one step command with gesture).

AR9 H: Does your child point to at least one body part on command?

Figure C-9, cont'd

AR9 T: Have mother command baby, "Show me your . . ." or "Where's your . . ." without pointing to the desired part herself.

AR10 H: Can child do two things in a row if asked? For example, "First go get your shoes, then sit down."

AR10 T: Set out ball, cup, and spoon and say, "*(Child's name)*, give me the spoon, then give the ball to mommy." Use slow, steady voice but do *not* break command into two separate sentences. If no response, *then* give each half of command separately to see if child understands separate components. If child succeeds on at least half of command, then give each of the following: "*(Child's name)*, give me the ball and give mommy the spoon." May repeat once, but do not break into two commands. Then, "Give mommy the ball, then give the cup to me." Pass if at least two two-step commands executed correctly. (Note: Child is credited even if the order of execution of a command is reversed.)

AR11 H: Place a cup, ball, and spoon on the table. Command child, "Show me/where is/give me the . . . cup/ball/spoon." (If command is "Give me," be sure to replace each object before asking about the next object.) Pass = two items correctly identified.

AR12 T: Put cup, ball, spoon, and crayon on table and give command, "Show me/where is/give me . . . the one we drink with/eat with/draw (color, write) with/throw (play with)." If the command "Give me" is used, be sure to replace each object before asking about the next object. Pass = two or more objects correctly identified.

AR13: Put out cup (upside down) and a 1-inch red cube. Command the child, "Put the block underneath the cup". Repeat × 1 on × 2 if necessary. If no attempt or if incorrect response, then demonstrate correct reponse, saying, "See now the block is *underneath* the cup." Remove the block and hand it to the child. Then give command, "Put the block *on top* of the cup." If child makes no response, then repeat command × 1 but do *not* demonstrate. Then command, "Put the block *behind* the cup," then "Put the block *beside* the cup." Pass = two or more commands correctly executed (*before* demonstration by examiner, if "underneath" is scored).

Figure C-9, cont'd

IV. Visual

VI H: "Does your baby smile for you? Not just a gas bubble or a burp, but a real smile?"

VI T: Have mother attempt to elicit smile by any means.

V2 H: "Does your baby seem to recognize you, reacting differently to you than to the sight of other people? For example, does your baby smile more quickly for you than for other people?"

V3 H: "Does your baby seem to recognize any common objects by sight? For example (if bottle or spoon fed), what happens when bottle or spoon is brought into view but *before* it touches baby's lips?" Pass if baby gets visibly excited or opens mouth in anticipation of feeding.

V4 H: "Does your baby respond to your facial expressions?"

V4 T: Engage baby's gaze and attempt to elicit a smile by smiling and talking to baby. Then scowl at baby. Pass if any change in baby's facial expression.

V5 T: Horizontal (H): Engage child's gaze with yours at a distance of 18 inches. Move slowly back and forth. Pass if child turns head 60° to the left and right from midline. Vertical (V): Move slowly up and down. Pass if child elevates eyes 30° from horizontal. Must pass both H and V to pass item.

V6 T: Flick your fingers rapidly toward child's face, ending with fingertips 1 to 2 inches from face. Do not touch face or eyelashes. Pass if child blinks.

V7 H: Does child play pat-a-cake, peek-a-boo, etc., in response to parents?

V8 T: See note for AR8 (always try AR8 first; if AR8 is passed, then automatically give credit for V8).

V9 H: Does child spontaneously initiate gesture games?

V10 H: "Does your child ever point with index finger to something wanted? For example, if child is sitting at the dinner table and wants something that is out of reach, how does child let you know what is wanted?" Pass *only* index finger pointing, *not* reaching with whole hand.

Figure C-9, cont'd

Early Language Milestone Scale (ELM Scale)
Update—June 1987

The Early Language Milestone Scale (ELM Scale) was introduced into clinical practice in 1983. Since that time, the ELM Scale has been used successfully in a variety of settings, including well-child clinics, neonatal intensive care follow-up programs, public school screening programs, and doctors' offices. The purpose of this communication is to acquaint you with one significant addition and several minor revisions that have recently been incorporated into the Auditory Expressive division of the ELM Scale.

The biggest change has been the addition of a new item cluster pertaining to intelligibility of speech. The Auditory Expressive division of the ELM Scale now consists of two parts: Content (cooing, babbling, use of words, phrases, etc.) and Intelligibility. This Intelligibility Cluster has been added in response to requests from users of the ELM Scale because many children seen for evaluation of "delayed speech" have unclear (unintelligible) speech.

Administration of Intelligibility Cluster
The Intelligibility Cluster
contains three bars: AE15: "About half"
                         AE19: "Three quarters"
                         AE20: "All or almost all"

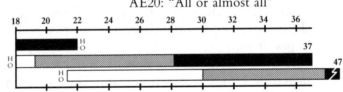

All three items may be scored by asking the parent the following forced-choice question:

"How clear is your child's speech? That is, how much of your child's speech can a stranger understand: Less than half, about half, three quarters, or all or almost all?"

Parents or other adults in close contact with a child often become attuned to the child's speech pattern, including any distortions of speech-sound production. Parents, therefore, are *not* the best ones to judge the intelligibility of their own child's speech. This is why the parent is asked to guess how clear the child sounds to *others:* "How much of your child's speech can a *stranger* understand. . .?" The wording *must* be followed when eliciting the parent's response.

Scoring
If parents report that "less than half" of the child's speech can be understood by strangers: child fails all three items in Intelligibility Cluster.

If "about half" of child's speech can be understood by strangers: child

Figure C-10

passes AE15 ("about half") but fails AE19 ("three quarters") and AE20 ("all or almost all").

If "three quarters" of child's speech can be understood by strangers: child passes both AE15 ("about half") and AE19 ("three quarters") but fails AE20 ("all or almost all").

If "all or almost all" of child's speech can be understood by strangers: child passes all three items in Intelligibility Cluster.

If the child fails to attain intelligibility at a level equal to that already attained by 90% or more of children of the same age, then the child fails the Intelligibility Cluster and the ELM Scale as a whole.

When to Administer the Intelligibility Cluster

The Intelligibility Cluster should be administered to all children 18 months of age or older. It should be administered *in addition* to the three or more items required to obtain a basal level in the Content portion of the Auditory Expressive division. A child over the age of 18 months must pass both the Intelligibility Cluster *and* the Content portion of the Auditory Expressive division to pass the Auditory Expressive division as a whole.

Special Cases

1. Some children over the age of 18 months may not be scoreable in the Intelligibility Cluster because they are not producing any words, intelligible or otherwise. Such children all fail the ELM Scale because of their delay in the appearance of speech, since the 90% value for the emergence of single words is approximately 17.5 months.

2. The primary age range of the ELM Scale is from birth to 36 months. Note that the 90% value for item AE19 is 37 months, and for item AE20, 47 months. Since the ELM Scale is often used with children over 36 months whose speech or language are delayed, these age values are displayed for convenience at the right hand edge of the bar for these two items.

Other Revisions to ELM Scale

Two items have been eliminated: old item AE15 (correct use of "me" and "you") and old item AE19 (correct use of the pronoun "I"). This should produce minimal effect on scoring: Old item AE15 (correct use of "me" and "you") was represented by a place holder on the first edition of the ELM Scale and was not used in scoring the Scale. The 90% value for old item AE19 (correct use of the pronoun "I") extended well above 36 months of age. Therefore, the child's performance on this item was unlikely to determine whether the child passed or failed the ELM Scale as a whole. Note that the item *numbers* AE15 and AE19 have been reassigned to two of the three bars in the Intelligibility Cluster. All of the other Auditory Expressive items stay in the same sequence as on the first edition of the ELM Scale, with same number designations as before.

Figure C-10, cont'd

Index